WISDOM FROM THE HOMELESS

Lessons a doctor learned at a homeless shelter

NEIL CRATON M.D.

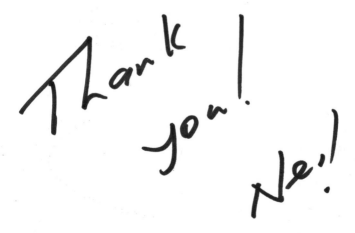

Thank you!

Neil!

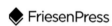 FriesenPress

Suite 300 - 990 Fort St
Victoria, BC, V8V 3K2
Canada

www.friesenpress.com

ISBN
978-1-5255-3137-8 (Hardcover)
978-1-5255-3138-5 (Paperback)
978-1-5255-3139-2 (eBook)

1. Body, Mind & Spirit, Inspiration & Personal Growth

Distributed to the trade by The Ingram Book Company

TABLE OF CONTENTS

ACKNOWLEDGMENT

The photographs in this book were taken by Leah Denbok and published in the work, *Nowhere to Call Home; Photographs and Stories of the Homeless, Volume One,* as well as her website, ldenbokphotography.com. They are not images of any characters described in this book nor of other patrons of Siloam Mission. I have included these images because they capture the essence of the men and women I have met there and they communicate the wide range of emotions one encounters in homeless people. Many thanks to Leah and her dad, Tim, for generously allowing me to use them.

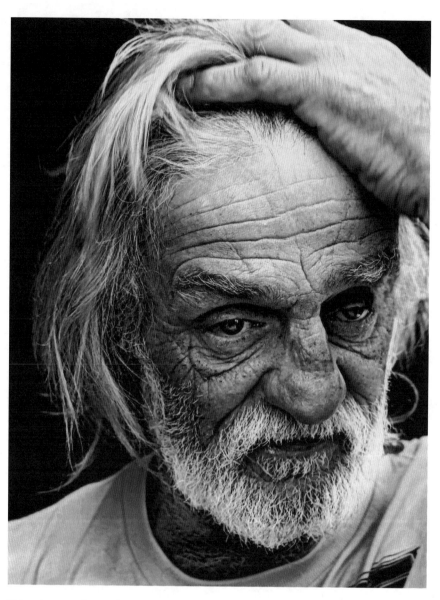

This photograph is taken with permission from Leah Denbok's work, *Nowhere to Call Home. Photographs and Stories of the Homeless. Volume One* or her website. It is not an image of any character referred to in this book. To see more of Leah's photography, visit ldenbokphotography.com.

DEDICATION

This book is dedicated to Siloam Mission.

A place of hope, healing, kindness, mercy, love and ultimately, unexpected wisdom.

All proceeds from the sale of this book will go to support the work done there.

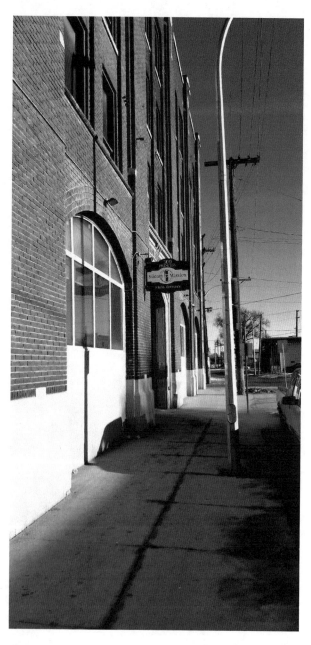

This photograph was taken by me on a beautiful Friday morning heading into the Mission.

PREFACE

Sometimes the world seems like a very dark place. Partisan grievances have increased exponentially. Left and Right find new ways to vilify each other, hardening points of view into the points of a spear. To disagree with someone is to hate them. A news cycle is not complete without a tragic tale of someone killing their neighbor or themselves. Children are terrified that the planet is ecologically doomed, where every breath of wind is perceived as the first whisper of the apocalypse. We are increasingly fearful of one another, drowning in a toxic soup of racial tension, political gamesmanship, ethnic marginalization and the vicious habit of "depersonalizing everyone into a rival." (1) The affluent seem increasingly obsessed with "small minded and lop-sided pursuits." (1) Now more than ever, we are suffering from a deficiency of kindness and hope.

In this dark and angry world, I see a glimpse of light. I have seen kindness, care and hope at a homeless Mission. In the spiritual tradition of this Mission, the source for hope, light, care and kindness is Jesus of Nazareth. The Mission, Siloam, is named after an ancient pool referred to in the gospel of John, where Jesus healed a person. In this tradition, the Mission has a medical clinic, and I have had the privilege of working there.

Hope for healing may be the most important benefit doctors can give to their patients. People of all walks of life need hope and every problem is easier to handle if we have it. Hope is hard to serve without the garnish of kindness. The present cultural context seems to know little of kindness. I have witnessed far more hope and kindness at Siloam than I see in many celebrities, newscasters or politicians.

This book isn't about me. I'm not an activist. I don't go to protests, and I seldom engage politically. I have only reluctantly become an advocate. I would be lying if I said I was a champion of the homeless. This book also isn't about medicine. While all the lessons were learned in a medical context, I believe they represent wisdom for all.

This book is about homeless people. It is inspired by the incredibly difficult lives lived by men and women who attend a homeless mission in Winnipeg, Manitoba. This book is about joy that can be seen in the midst of that difficulty. It is about the powerful role suffering can have in shaping our character and our lives. It is about the overcoming of that suffering and the inspiration that comes from persevering through adversity. This book is about the wisdom that people with nothing can teach all of us in affluent North American culture. Ultimately, this book is about relationship—the type of relationships you can discover when you decide to serve your fellow man.

Telling a patient's story needs to be done with discretion and care as it always involves an act of appropriation. The physician is opening a closed door, looking into a soul, discovering truths that are profoundly personal. The telling of that story demands meticulous safeguards to protect the identity of the patient. (2) Yet, there are few things more meaningful to doctors than the stories of their patients. Danielle Ofri, a physician-writer and scholar, notes that when she began writing her book, *What Doctors Feel: How Emotions Affect the Practice of Medicine*, she asked her medical colleagues to tell her what made them the doctor they are today. (3) She was flooded with responses, and not one physician mentioned Harrison's *Textbook of Internal Medicine*, *The Lancet*, or any disease process. Instead, they related meaningful stories inspired by their patients. Ofri observed that the stories were crafted with metaphor, character development, irony, connection, interpretation and perspective – skills more reflective of the humanities than the biomedical sciences. This makes sense, since doctors are immersed in their patient's stories, tales of tragedy and victory, suffering and perseverance, pain and joy. Ofri found that doctors often have profound emotional reactions to the work they do, and she concluded that exploration of these reactions may offer benefit to the patient, doctors and society at large. (4)

A respectful rendering of a patient's story should honor them and what they've endured. If a particular story can edify future physicians, or the public, there is value in sharing it. (4) These are my hopes in relating these stories: to honor the homeless patients I have seen at Siloam; to acknowledge all they have endured; to provide some of benefit to young doctors and to raise awareness of the overwhelming challenges faced by this group of people.

The stories in this book are true. Only one patient's story was fictionalized into a hybrid of several people to ensure anonymity of the character. To protect the patients' identities, I have changed all names and most of the genders, ages, races and physical characteristics of the individuals. Any medical condition that would allow the identification of a patient has been altered. I have not changed the ethnic background of the Indigenous patients, as the suffering faced by Indigenous people in Canada is very real and needs to be contemplated by a wide audience. I have learned that referring to an Indigenous person by their tribal origin is honorable. Unfortunately, at the time of my encounters with these Indigenous people, I was unaware of that fact, and so failed to ask my patients of their tribal origins.

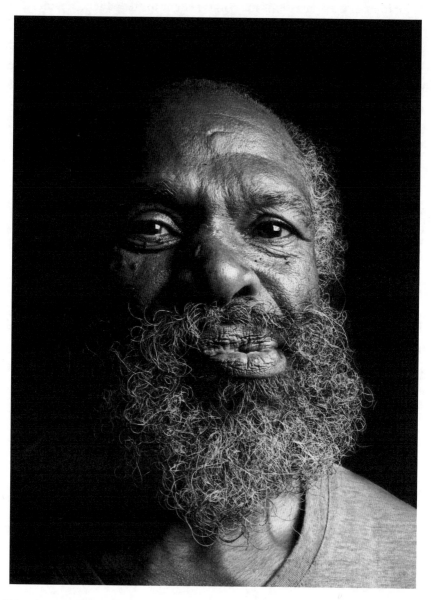

This photograph is taken with permission from Leah Denbok's work, *Nowhere to Call Home. Photographs and Stories of the Homeless. Volume One* or her website. It is not an image of any character referred to in this book. To see more of Leah's photography, visit ldenbokphotography.com.

INTRODUCTION

I held the bloodied head in my hands, careful not to move the man's neck. The profound muscle tension and violent movements of his arms and legs were subsiding. I could see, hear and feel that this man was able to move air, despite his labored breathing and compromised airway. The smell of his breath was crudely intoxicating, probably a combination of rubbing alcohol and vomit. Blood trickled from his mouth and from a laceration over his left eye. The cut was laid on a bed of countless prior scars—the face of a fighter? His nose had been broken several times, and leaned a bit to the right, looking to be on sentinel duty for rest of the poor man's face. Only two or three teeth remained in his mouth, and they looked precarious. I had about 200 spectators as I stabilized the man's spine and airway. The onlookers were a diverse cast of concerned characters, a group of homeless people I had come to know and care for. This man was probably having an alcohol-withdrawal seizure, and I had answered a call for help.

I was working in the medical clinic at a homeless shelter in Winnipeg, Manitoba. The man had experienced the seizure while waiting for lunch and collapsed in the food line. People were understandably frightened, as a grand mal seizure is quite a spectacle for the uninitiated. The patient loses consciousness, makes deep guttural noises, froths at the mouth and has intense and rhythmic movements of their extremities. In Biblical times, sufferers of grand mal seizures were thought to be possessed by demons.

We had called 911 and an ambulance was on its way. My patient had an acceptable heart rate and palpable blood pressure, which indicated he was not in any immediate danger. The witnesses watched carefully and I adjusted his jaw to maintain his airway. Kneeling at the man's head, cradling his troubled face in my arms, in the food line of a homeless shelter, surrounded by homeless people and Mission volunteers, it felt surreal. As we waited for the ambulance I wondered: "How did the two of us get here?" I was a typical middle-aged, white professional with a wife, two kids and a house in the suburbs. His journey was obviously much more difficult.

I grew up in a home with substantial dysfunction. My parents met and were married in World War II and were never really suited for each other. I believe that my dad had undiagnosed post-traumatic stress disorder—PTSD—having been shot down in a Lancaster Bomber over Germany during the war. The captain, he lost 10 members of his crew of 12. He medicated his PTSD with alcohol, a plight common in veterans. My mother didn't navigate the alcohol use well; my dad had originally intended to be a pastor, a goal that was lost among the empty bottles. A death in our family would be the final straw that hardened their hearts toward each other. I felt like a pawn in their relationship, the only child still at home, being used in their attempts to hurt and embarrass one another. My impression of family life was that it was filled with pain, anguish and embarrassment. I would hold onto this impression for years.

Outside the home, I think the best description of me was that I was a jock. Athletics provided a wonderful diversion from life at home. I loved all sports and became fairly good at basketball and football. I was fortunate enough to be selected a city all-star for both sports in my final year of high school. Later, I became an endurance athlete, and completed three Ironman triathlons and 15 marathons. Fitness and good health were my passions.

In high school, I dated a girl who, ironically, introduced me to the woman who is now my wife. My girlfriend's family had a cottage in the lake country close to our city, and I absolutely loved being with them in that environment. They gave me hope that family life could be joyful and uncomplicated by anger, bitterness and strife. I had a great group high school friends, many of whom I still enjoy today. We were full of pranks and many hijinx followed us on our journeys together. I am proud to have been the charter member of the CIA, "Craton's Immature Army." I suspect we were "over-fond of the grape", as most of our activities centered around beer. One crazy long weekend at a National Park in our province saw several of us in the back of a Royal Canadian Mounted Police cruiser for conduct that the officers characterized as "somewhat unruly." We actually made it as far as the local jail where my tipsy co-defendant named the province's Justice Minister as his next-of-kin.

So just how did I find myself serving at a mission for the homeless, on my knees, protecting the neck and airway of an Indigenous man having an alcohol withdrawal seizure? Let me try to connect the dots.

My journey to a homeless mission starts with Jesus. I first encountered his teachings in 1980, when I was 21 years old. I had begun my first year of medical school. I had fallen in love with a beautiful woman and (spoiler alert) she is now my wife.

Kate was from a strong Christian family. Early in our relationship, we were at a party when a friend of hers told me that this wonderful woman would never marry me because I was not a Christian. I was shocked, first because I thought Kate wanted to marry me, but also because I thought I *was* a Christian. I assumed that anyone born in Canada was a Christian, unless of course you were Jewish. Obviously, my theology was not well-established. Even though my family of origin issues had convinced me that marriage was the last institution I wanted to be part of, I was disgruntled that Kate wouldn't marry me. She would have to explain herself. That evening, in the most hypothetical of contexts, I put the question to her: Kate, would you marry me? The answer was honest and difficult to hear. Apparently, being "unequally yoked" (an expression I would remember well) to a person who didn't share her Christian faith mattered to Kate.

I was like most 20 year-old guys—interested in sports, women, partying with my friends, personal gratification and career advancement. Having been admitted into medical school, I thought my future was set. I was determined to convince Kate that she could consider marriage to someone who did not share her faith. It would all work out in the end. Little did I know.

Kate and I had a magical summer in 1980. The weather was spectacular with an endless string of warm sunny days. I had bought a rusty old Porsche 914 hard top convertible for $2500 and we travelled around the province in any free time we had, singing and laughing together. Trips to the beach with the top down and a blossoming romance make for fond memories. A good friend and I had a landscaping business, and we had some control of our work hours, so I tried to see Kate as much as possible, despite the poorly-fitting yoke.

One hot August weekend we were at a lake cabin with a bunch of friends in the dog days of summer. The cabin was on the beautiful Lake of the Woods, one of the most wonderful fresh water lakes in the world. We were having a great time frolicking in the water, hanging out, jumping off the boathouse, enjoying the pristine lake with dozens of friends. In the midst of the frivolity, I experienced an unusual conviction. I felt a strong desire to go to church with Kate. I had no idea where the inclination came from and was hesitant to share it with her. I tried to compartmentalize the thought, but it seemed to push its way to the front of my mind. I floated the idea out to Kate. She was definitely caught off-guard and seemed flustered. Somewhat reluctantly, she agreed we could drive in from the lake early and go to an evening church service back in Winnipeg. I had no idea why we were doing this and no idea what God had planned.

Kates' home church had no evening service that day, so she picked a Pentecostal church in the downtown of Winnipeg, our moderate size mid-western city. I was very nervous as we neared the facility, regretting my moment of inspiration. I hadn't been in a church for at least a decade. I peppered Kate with questions as we approached our destination. Would there be any fanatics in this place? Would they speak in tongues or perform secret rituals? Would they know that I was a pagan? Through all my paranoid ruminations, Kate assured me that I would be just fine. I didn't have to do anything, just listen and be quiet.

The building was much larger than churches I was used to, and it probably sat 3000 people. The overall vibe was quite interesting, with a diverse crowd of New Canadians, Indigenous people and Caucasians of all ages. I was surprised how many people were there on a hot summer night. The singing of the faithful was actually kind of nice. The pastor was a model of rectitude, a good speaker, very articulate and engaging. To my surprise, I was actually enjoying my first adult church experience. Maybe Kate was on to something. My joy was short-lived.

My jaw hit the floor when the sermon title was announced. The topic of the message, on that hot August night, was the peril to Christians of being married to those who didn't follow Jesus—the dreaded "unequally yoked." The pastor now seemed like my mortal enemy, as he recited the dangers of relationships with people like me, particularly for young people in love. Biblical scripture was read to corroborate his position. (5) This would surely convince Kate to end this unequal yoking once and for all. Our relationship was doomed. I became increasingly uncomfortable and wanted desperately to escape the sanctuary before Kate made any final decisions about us. The only problem was my legs wouldn't move.

Eventually the pastor began wrapping things up. The crowd started to sing the hymn "Just as I Am." (6) I didn't know the song, but it is very familiar to churchgoers who have witnessed an altar call. If you have ever watched a Billy Graham crusade, you have probably seen one. The presenter gives those in the crowd an invitation to make a public commitment to follow Jesus by coming down to the altar. I had never experienced anything like this, and it unfolded in a most memorable fashion.

The sermon was finally over and I started to relax. Kate didn't seem to be withdrawing from my side. The words of the hymn were definitely resonating with me. I wanted to be accepted by Kate (and God), "just as I am." And so, when the pastor asked us to bow our heads and invited us to raise our hands if we wanted him to pray for us, I tentatively put up my hand. What harm could come from this nice old man praying for me in my vulnerable state of debauchery and asymmetric yoking? The prayer might also help Kate with her deliberations.

The pastor seemed to acknowledge my hand in the air with a "Yes, thank you in the balcony" although I barely cleared the top of my head with my sweaty palm. But when the prayer ended and I opened my eyes and raised my head, the pastor made an astonishing request. "Thank you all for responding to the Lord. I now invite all of you who raised your hands to come down to the altar and do your business with Jesus." My business with Jesus? *My business with Jesus?* My business was with Kate, not this fanatical pastor, and certainly not Jesus. My mood swung from slightly nervous to utterly paranoid. What kind of crazy cult was this? What had I gotten myself into? We could still be at the lake! I certainly was not going down to the altar on the main floor of this cavernous auditorium. Even if I had wanted to go, my legs still wouldn't move. Finally, the hymn ended. I was amazed to see a large contingent of people surrounding the altar, some smiling, some weeping, others accompanied by loved ones. The pastor then justified my paranoia and singled me out, with a personalized invitation to the altar: "There is one more up in the balcony, you know who you are. We are going to sing another verse of "Just as I am", just for you ... Please join us here at the altar and come to Jesus. You know who you are."

Kate turned and looked at me, horrified, part fear, part incredulity, her eyes pleading for reassurance that I hadn't done what she feared. I nodded, sweat dripping from my forehead: oh yes, this was for me. I grabbed her hand and we headed for the exit; my legs would just have to follow with the rest of me. A powerful force was at work inside me, and I had no clue what it was. All I knew was that this pastor was not going to get me into his cult, and that we had to get out of that building! I honestly feared that the doors might be locked as we raced out of the sanctuary. I needed a beer.

Kate and I went to local restaurant to review the fiasco. I was still feeling very tense, with adrenaline stoking my heart and making me tremble. My agitation began to abate, as it appeared none of the zealots had followed us out of the sanctuary. We talked, we laughed, and it seemed as if Kate still liked me. Maybe we wouldn't be breaking our yoke, at least not that night.

Upon reflection, this was probably my first memorable encounter with what Christians call the Holy Spirit. Kate's elder sister suggested I start reading the Gospel of John and just see what I found. In Jesus, I encountered the most wonderful person, a man of compassion and wisdom. A man of contemplation and action. A man of love, who was not afraid to challenge the establishment or the status quo. This man seemed like a liberator of women, and a friend to the poor. He was a healer and a miracle worker. The man was the Light of the World, and the way, the truth and the life. I wanted to become a follower of this man, but felt as if I didn't measure up, having too many problems and shortcomings in my life. Kate's sister again helped me through the impasse, advising that I didn't have to "clean myself up" to follow Jesus. She explained that getting rid of my baggage would be a lifelong process. I just had to believe and receive. Well, I believed and received and started down a new path. After a few months of reading the Gospels and discussing things with Kate and her family, I simply decided to follow Jesus.

That decision took my life in a new direction, but I never expected that following Jesus would lead me to a homeless shelter, some 30 years later. I began a personal journey where I would learn the truth about Jesus as savior and Lord, and my need to develop a meaningful relationship with Him. While I acknowledge that many will not share this path or this commitment, the lessons in this book are based on that foundation and are, I believe, of universal application. I hope that you will be able to read these stories about homeless people, even if you have a different belief system.

The idea to provide medical care at a homeless shelter came from an unexpected source. His name was Abe and he was an octogenarian physician. He and his wife were founding members of the church that Kate attended. He seemed like most retired men—quiet, proper, reserved. Having just been admitted to medical school, I was interested in physicians' lives. What was it like being a doctor? Do they like their work? Do they have any time for their families or recreation? Do they seem content with their career path? Abe didn't answer any of these questions for me because I was too afraid to ask him; like most guys, I don't ask anyone for advice. However, I learned through a friend that Abe, despite being close to 90, was still looking after patients at a Salvation Army shelter. I was moved by this, and always remember the respect I felt for this quiet man. Providing care for a group of people with nothing, who often don't get a fair shake from society seemed so kind. This was magnified by the fact that the servant was a little old man. If he could do it, couldn't I? Shouldn't I? It would take me many years to respond to that call.

My preparation for work at a homeless shelter came through my tenure at the largest emergency department in Winnipeg. From 1986 to 1990,

I worked at the Health Sciences Center. The Primary Health Care Unit saw all the patients who came to emergency not requiring an IV or a heart monitor. We also provided primary health care to patients who had tertiary care problems. For example, we would provide basic medical care to those on dialysis and those who had received an organ transplant. One of our major constituencies was the homeless population, often Indigenous, addicted and mentally ill. I learned to respect these people through their struggles and felt a definite affinity for them. The practice of medicine with this complex group of patients provided many challenges. A lack of social supports, poor compliance, the ravages of addiction, terrible food and unpredictable shelter make these people uniquely vulnerable. By working in this environment for several years, I learned how to interact with the homeless and treat their medical problems, while acknowledging that they are people who need a helping hand.

The final push I needed to start working at a homeless shelter came when a local mission was given a $1 Million endowment from the estate of a prominent pharmacist. Saul Sair bequeathed that substantial sum to Siloam Mission for the construction of a medical clinic in their facility.

The Mission is set in the heart of the toughest area of Winnipeg. Many shelters provide life-saving care to the homeless in this region. Siloam is one of the largest, providing beds for over 100 people every night. The Mission is situated in a five-story reclaimed brick warehouse. Its staff and volunteers provide three meals a day, clothes, counseling services and programs designed to get people into their own accommodation and eventually find a job. The addition of the clinic allowed the Mission to provide medical care, dentistry, physiotherapy, nursing, chiropractic, optometric and massage therapy services. When the clinic was opening and receiving substantial media attention, the passion of the clinic director was evident. She was interviewed by a local television station and shown to be a charismatic, energetic and altruistic young woman, clearly looking to make a difference in the lives of the people the Mission served. Her passion convicted me in some way, helping me to finally respond to the prompting that had been niggling inside of me for so many years . . . I was supposed to serve these people.

I called Carrie, the director, and went for a tour of Siloam and its clinic. I was blown away by the place. The clinic was beautifully designed and had all the necessary equipment to provide a diverse offering of health care services. The staff and volunteers were enthusiastic, and a sense of joy, purpose, and commitment filled the place. I was convinced that I should be working there too. I signed up for a shift and became part of the team. I would try and serve every second Friday morning. It seemed that God was working there, and I wanted to get involved.

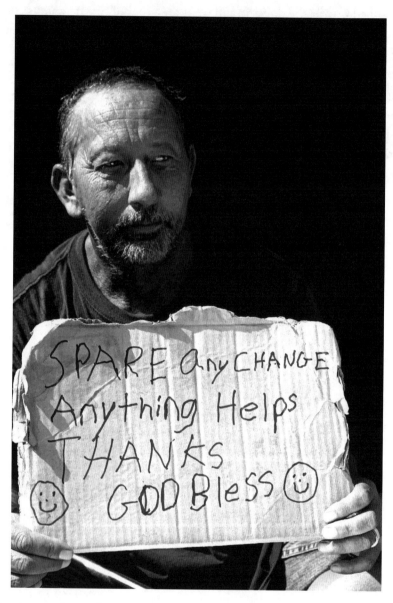

This photograph is taken with permission from Leah Denbok's work, *Nowhere to Call Home. Photographs and Stories of the Homeless. Volume One* or her website. It is not an image of any character referred to in this book. To see more of Leah's photography, visit ldenbokphotography.com.

A BRIEF LOOK AT SILOAM MISSION

Siloam Mission is named after a pool described in the Gospel of John in which Jesus healed a blind man. (7) Remnants of the pool of Siloam have been discovered by modern-day archaeologists, close to old Jerusalem. Siloam Mission is set in an area that was once a thriving neighborhood, back in the early 1900's when Winnipeg vied to be a city on par with Chicago. The area is on the southern edge of Winnipeg's widely-known "North End." This core area now has a reputation for poverty, crime, violence and racial divides. It is in this milieu that the Mission strives to be a connecting point between the compassionate and Winnipeg's less fortunate. Siloam Mission is a Christian humanitarian organization that alleviates hardships and provides opportunities for change for those affected by homelessness. As a faith-based and faith-operated organization, the Mission treats all people as objects of God's love, mercy and grace, and who deserve to be treated with dignity and respect. Compassion is seen as an expression of God's care and love for hungry, homeless and hurting people. Siloam believes in networking with people of all walks of life, and that volunteers are vital. The Mission works with other inner-city agencies and ministries to help the homeless and those in the neighborhood who are affected by poverty.

Compassion is the emotion most commonly ascribed to Jesus in the New Testament. "When he saw the crowds, he had compassion for them, because they were harassed and helpless, like sheep without a shepherd." (8) This description would fit most of those using Siloam Mission's services. Many of the clients who attend seem without direction, harassed by mental illness and addiction, feeling without help and without hope.

The Greek word used to describe the compassion of Jesus is "splagchnon." The term "splanchnic" is a medical reference to the human gut. The word is best translated as a movement in the inward parts, a sort of visceral reaction. Scholars have taken this to mean that the compassion of Jesus is not merely intellectual or cognitive. It is a deep inner stirring in one's gut that leads to action. For close to 30 years, I had a cognitive and intellectual compassion for homeless people, but it wasn't until I began working at the Mission that I could say it was "splanchnic", something that stirred in my gut and lead to action. Most people working at the Mission seem to be motivated by this visceral type of compassion. It is rewarding to work with people who are "moved to action."

The epidemic of homelessness is a relatively recent development in Canada.

In the late 1980's, homelessness became much more common as a consequence of a reduction in government investment in affordable housing coupled with a sharp decrease in full time employment. There was also reduced spending on social and health supports all across the country. By the year 2000, 235,000 people per year were homeless, and over 35,000 on any given night. (9) It seems as though our society has chosen homelessness.

Historically, homelessness was the plight of single men but as the homeless population grew, so did its diversity. Youth, families, Indigenous Peoples, newcomers, refugees and individuals identifying as LGBTQ all became more likely to find themselves on the streets. Homelessness became more visible by the sheer number of individuals on Canadian streets with no home to return to. Indigenous Peoples in particular face significant barriers to affordable housing and are disproportionately represented in the homeless population, particularly in urban centers. While making up only 4.3% of the general population, Indigenous Peoples account for up to 35% of the homeless. Indigenous Peoples' experiences of poverty and homelessness are firmly rooted in colonial practices and systemic discrimination. (9) These demographic features certainly seem to apply at Siloam.

Between 2010 and 2014, an estimated 450,000 Canadians used a homeless shelter at least once. Most shelter stays were short term, on average less than 10 days for youth and adults. For some groups, the length of stay has increased considerably. In particular, seniors (50+) and families stay more than 20 days on average. The length of stay for all types of shelter-users increased between 2005 and 2014. I have seen patients at Siloam who have *lived* there for over a year. The use of emergency shelters by seniors has nearly doubled in the last decade. It is particularly sad to see an old timer limp into the Mission clinic, cane in one hand, back pack with all his or her worldly belongings in the other. Unfortunately, the evidence indicates this is becoming more common. (9)

Even though the data suggests that the number of people using shelters has decreased since 2005, the number of beds occupied on any given night has actually increased between 2010 and 2014. In addition, the number of stays lasting 30 days or more increased to 12% in 2014. Another worrisome feature is that close to 95% of all shelter beds across the country are full every night. The strain on shelter capacity, and the fact that the average number of bed nights per person has increased, suggest we are not responding as effectively as we need to in order to move people out of homelessness.

Homeless people, especially those with addictions and mental health problems, can be housed and cared for, but finding permanent, safe, clean and independent places to live remains elusive. The ultimate goal of organizations like Siloam is for all people to have their own place to live, with all the benefits and dignity this can bring. Unless our culture decides that these people are worth our investment, I fear that we will continue to need homeless shelters.

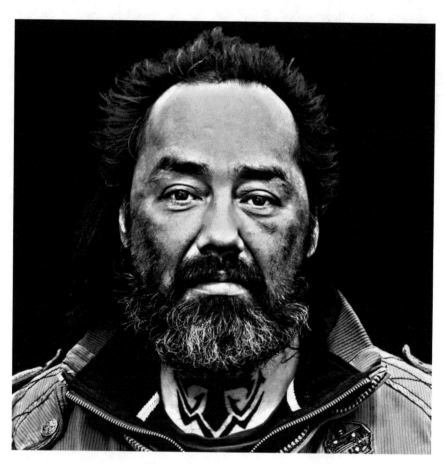

This photograph is taken with permission from Leah Denbok's work, *Nowhere to Call Home. Photographs and Stories of the Homeless. Volume One* or her website. It is not an image of any character referred to in this book. To see more of Leah's photography, visit ldenbokphotography.com.

LESSON 1:   Sometimes silent screams are the loudest.

Prayer in action is love, and love in action is service. Try to give unconditionally whatever a person needs in the moment . . . Do not worry about why problems exist in the world – just respond to people's needs.
—Mother Teresa

There is a passage in the New Testament which highlights a remarkable technique for changing one's perspective in dealing with a difficult situation. (10) In the gospel story of Matthew 25, Jesus describes two types of people: those who serve people in need (referred to as sheep) and those who don't (called goats). He lists many types of people who need help - the hungry, the naked, those in prison, the sick and strangers - exactly the sort of people you meet at Siloam. Jesus says that whenever we serve "the least of these brothers" of His, we actually serve Him. There is reward for the sheep, judgment for the goats. Apparently, Jesus wanted his followers to care for those who had experienced suffering, loss, rejection and failure. The lesson of the sheep and the goats always resonated with me and helped me work in the city center emergency department earlier in my career. It would prove even more helpful dealing with a poor, silent man, on a cold winter night, in one of my first shifts at the Mission.

The people one meets in a homeless shelter usually look rough around the edges. Second hand clothing and a limited ability to bathe lead to a characteristic, tussled appearance. The patient I was about to see had the usual tattered attire, but his facial features were remarkable. In fact, I wondered if he was an actor playing a part. He was an Indigenous man in his early thirties with a chiseled jaw and shimmering black hair cascading below his shoulders, hair that could have come straight out of a shampoo commercial. It seemed so incongruous with the rest of his presentation. The paradox was intensified by how badly he smelled. I caught the distinct odor associated with glue-sniffing, as well as the recognizable smell of anaerobic bacterial infection. His demeanor was similarly remarkable. He didn't speak. Despite his silence, I could tell he was listening to everything I said and I began my medical evaluation. He appeared lucid, followed instructions and was extraordinarily calm. There were no entries in his chart indicating any medical history. He refused a paper and pen. He appeared surprisingly well-muscled. I asked him how I could help him and he nodded towards a temporary cast on his left arm. I asked him what he had done, and he just nodded toward the brace. He wasn't keen on answering any other questions, so I asked him if I could remove the cast and have a look. He nodded again.

As I approached him, the unmistakable odor of a dangerous bacteria known as pseudomonas aeruginosa was present. The smell is well known to health care providers who work with patients in difficult situations. This type of bacteria often infects compromised hosts and is always trouble. The man's temporary cast was saturated with blood and pus. I had to moisten the wrapping to remove it. It looked like it had been stuck to his arm for days. It was this act of removing his splint, with all its odor, blood and purulent material that brought to mind the words of Jesus in Matthew 25: "What you do for the least of these, you do for me." (10) This man needed mercy not judgment. I tried to imagine that I held the hand of Jesus, and for me that transformed the moment into something transcendent. I was no longer fighting through the smell of glue and infection or trying to figure out how this man got here; I was meeting God.

Once the splint was off, it was apparent that my patient had major problems. The skin was open and infected, and his wrist was so badly broken that the bones moved freely. My silent patient was suffering from an infected, unstable and open fracture that had been unattended for days.

He needed to be treated surgically and required intravenous antibiotic coverage. I was worried he would lose his hand. I called the hospital emergency room and the orthopedic surgeon on call, and they agreed to see the man immediately. We sent him to the hospital by taxi and we confirmed his arrival at the hospital a few hours later.

During our entire interaction, the man never spoke to me. His rugged face, his perfect hair, the overpowering odor and his utter silence painted the most discordant picture. How did he get to this place and time? Did he simply choose not to speak? Why had he just surfaced for care now? These questions would go unanswered. I didn't want think of how this medical disaster came to be.

I have reflected on that experience many times. The idea that helping a person in need equates to helping Jesus is an amazing concept. That was the first of many times that I used that mental imagery prescribed by Jesus himself. It makes it an honor to look after "these brothers of [His]."

I thought I had seen the last of my silent patient as he slowly walked to the taxi, but about two months later he re-appeared at the clinic. His hair was still perfect, his face ruggedly handsome, but his left arm was amputated below the elbow. I asked him how I could help him, and he again nodded to his arm. We went through the same silent process and more trouble was to be found. The stump had become infected, and further medical intervention was required. He still didn't speak. He refused to write. He had no fixed address and no ID. The man's plight prompted so many haunting questions. What pain drove him to sniff glue? How can people like this silent man be helped? How can people with such obvious problems keep falling through the cracks? Questions like these are part of the fabric of the homeless world, the problems overwhelming, the solutions so inadequate. I tried to remind myself that I had been called to serve one person at a time and hoped others had been called to solve the larger systemic problems.

This man was probably one of the poor souls whose lives have been damaged by solvent abuse or sniffing glue. The sniffing of gas and glue by people on the street has profoundly negative consequences and is generally confined to the impoverished. It isn't something rich kids do.

The transient high is often followed by significant neurological damage and permanent cognitive impairment. This man's journey must have been profoundly painful.

The man endured his pain in silence. I remember feeling frustrated that there was so little I could do to change his situation. This man's case prompted me to consider the complicated convergence of societal forces driving people to the street. Substance abuse, poverty, mental illness and other pervasive problems can make one feel helpless. Faced with those emotions, I relied on the simple words of Jesus, "I was sick, and you looked after me."

I haven't seen the silent man since his second visit. I wonder if he is still alive. I wonder why he didn't speak. I think I can still hear him.

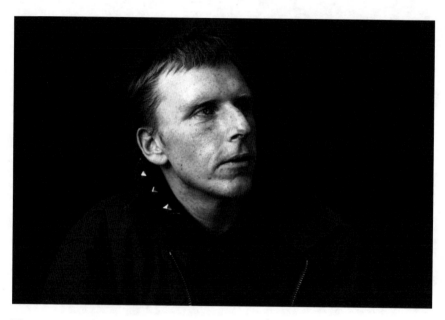

This photograph is taken with permission from Leah Denbok's work, *Nowhere to Call Home. Photographs and Stories of the Homeless. Volume One* or her website. It is not an image of any character referred to in this book. To see more of Leah's photography, visit ldenbokphotography.com.

LESSON 2: Kindness is a key. It opens hearts hardened by violence, minds shut by pain and spirits bound by condemnation.

Kindness is a language the deaf can hear and the blind can see.
—*Mark Twain*

It was a good morning. I was working with my twenty-year old niece, Rachel, who is like a daughter to me. She is smart and beautiful, and at the time was maintaining an A+ average in her second year of Science at the University of Winnipeg. Rachel was considering studying medicine and wanted to volunteer with me at Siloam. It was her first day, and we were seeing patients with basic medical problems. But even basic problems are complicated given the amazing individuals one encounters at a homeless shelter. The people who make up our homeless population usually have a powerful story to tell, often full of tragedy and heartache. Yet paradoxically, the stories often have elements of joy, strength, perseverance, victory and faith. There is a lot to learn from these people. Rachel was seeing the practice of medicine, but in an environment very different from her suburban home and with an unforgettable cast of characters.

Our last patient of the morning was a blind Metis man named Sam. He was in his early twenties and required a guide to help him make his way from the reception area to the examination room. He was tall and thin, neatly groomed, with a bright smile and a pleasant disposition. With his white cane folded on his lap, Sam informed us that he was hoping to be prescribed a drug to help regulate his sleep/wake cycle. Sam explained that blind people have a difficult time sleeping due to the lack of light fluctuation and its effect on humans' body-clock. Sam was in no rush and didn't seem to lose confidence when I told him that I had never heard of the drug he was requesting. I Googled the drug and confirmed there was such a product and it was available in Canada. After a few phone calls to local pharmacies, we learned that this was a special-order item, not carried in retail outlets due to the lack of demand. We were not going to be able to help Sam that day, but he lingered in the examination room. After a little small talk, Sam revealed some other significant concerns. I have found that patients in and out of the Mission often offer up an entrance complaint that doesn't reflect their real problem. After checking out the doc for the day and developing some trust, they then share their true difficulties.

Sam told us that he was regularly bullied and beaten. He was also hearing-impaired and had had his hearing aids stolen during a recent mugging on the streets of Winnipeg. This made his sight-impaired world nearly impossible to navigate. He had no money, and no chance of getting new hearing aids. He then shared another concern. He had a painful and swollen big toe but he couldn't see what was causing the pain. He didn't want to waste our time with a minor problem like a sore toe but he was really worried about it, as he had to be on his feet all day to avoid troubles on the street and the pain in the toe was affecting his gait.

Sam agreed to let us examine his toe. His sock was stuck to the skin, glued down by pus and dried blood. We wet the sock to allow it to be peeled off of his toe. We cleansed Sam's foot with saline and gauze. This foot-cleaning ritual is common at the Mission clinic, as homeless people's feet are jeopardized by poorly fitting shoes, damp socks and days spent walking to keep warm. I try to view the act of washing a homeless person's feet in the context of Jesus washing his disciples' feet. For me, this changes the experience from something clinical, to something sacred.

Sam's toe had a significant infection surrounding a damaged toenail. The toe was cherry red and under a great deal of pressure. He was soon to lose his nail, and I was worried about the integrity of the whole toe. Sam needed antibiotics and to have part of his toe nail removed to allow the infection to heal. The Mission carries a supply of common antibiotics so we can dispense them to people who have no means of paying for the medications. I decided to put Sam on a ten-day course of antibiotics and then have him to my regular clinic for removal of the toenail's infected edge. I wanted to give the antibiotics a chance to decrease the local infection before performing this mildly invasive procedure.

It was heartbreaking to hear Sam's next confession. As we put a dressing on his toe as gently as we could, Sam said no one had ever treated him with such kindness. I could tell Rachel was touched by his words and the whole experience with Sam. Seeing the difficulties that were part of his life, but also witnessing the joy and hope that still lived in his spirit, was a very powerful lesson. The types of difficulties Sam experienced helped Rachel and me realize the many things we take for granted. Safety, vision, hearing, a home, love from others, the simple kindness of our friends and family. There are so many gifts we don't consider, so many reasons to be thankful. The Mission staff were able to make arrangements for Sam to sleep there, and to come to my clinic later that week.

As we were saying our goodbyes, I asked our reception staff if Siloam had any contacts with hearing aid providers. While Rachel and I were finishing up our paperwork and discussing the day's cases, one of the women called a local audiology clinic to see if they could help out. To our amazement, the clinic owner offered to give Sam two brand new hearing aids on the spot. He just needed to get there. A bus ticket, provided by the Mission, got him on his way that very afternoon. Sam was rendered speechless by the news. He hugged us with tears streaming down his face. Sam referred to the events of the day as a miracle.

Sam was scheduled to come to my office the following Wednesday for removal of his toenail. I called the Mission when he failed to arrive. They informed me that Sam had taken a bus back to his home in Eastern Canada. He was fearful living on the streets in Winnipeg after his last beating but the trouble had been he had no money for a bus ticket back home. We learned that the audiologists were happy to help Sam get back to his home and had bought him a bus ticket to his town. We have never seen Sam again.

I sometimes wonder if Sam was an angel, sent to allow us to share in a *God moment*. For Rachel to have this experience, her first time working in a clinic, and her first time in a homeless mission setting, seemed more than coincidence. I am happy to report that Rachel is now in her first year of medical school. I think Sam taught her that kindness is something that opens hearts hardened by violence, minds shut by pain and spirits bound by condemnation.

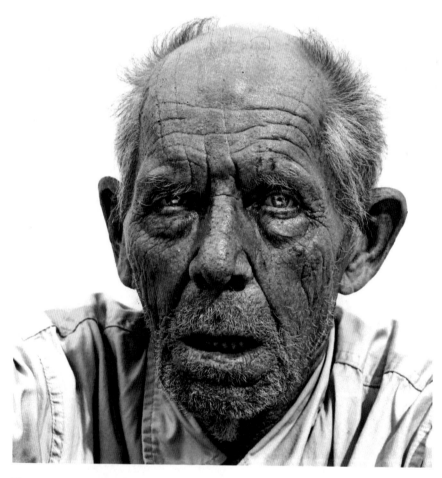

This photograph is taken with permission from Leah Denbok's work, *Nowhere to Call Home. Photographs and Stories of the Homeless. Volume One* or her website. It is not an image of any character referred to in this book. To see more of Leah's photography, visit ldenbokphotography.com.

LESSON 3: Empty bottles are the stuff of empty lives.

She's not getting drunk for the hell of it, she's getting drunk to numb the hell of it.
—Sean Bates

The destruction of human potential wrought by alcohol abuse is one of the most profound lessons that you learn working at a homeless shelter. It is well described in Proverbs 23, which paints a portrait of many of those we encounter at Siloam:

> Who has woe? Who has sorrow?
> Who has strife? Who has complaints?
> Who has needless bruises? Who has bloodshot eyes?
> Those who linger over wine (11).

Whatever relief might be gained by alcohol in the short term is far outweighed by the suffering it causes when used in excess and allowed to take over people's lives. I have always assumed that people abuse drugs and alcohol to escape troubles deep in their soul, to numb the hell and mask their grief, and the current evidence seems to support that notion.

Addiction and substance abuse are significant issues in the lives of many of the people who attend homeless missions. Our clients often find themselves in the epicenter of these tectonic forces, left to face the disastrous consequences of addiction which include poor health, fractured relationships, trouble with the law and poverty.

Historically, addiction has been viewed as a moral failing, a manifestation of a character defect or a lack of willpower. It has also been considered to be a disease process, in the classic bio-medical context. These models may be losing pre-eminence in the conceptualization of addiction. An emerging sociological framework recognizes that addiction is the avenue by which needy people respond to the lack of meaning and community in their lives. It is a complicated way of coping with traumatic events, dislocation, social fragmentation and isolation. Widespread dislocation is a negative consequence of our modern culture. Dislocation is defined as the absence of belonging, identity, meaning, and purpose. It flows from social fragmentation. Just as dislocation follows social fragmentation, addiction tends to follow dislocation. A large body of historical and anthropological evidence now shows the predictability of this sequence. (12)

When nothing else seems to be working, addiction can help dislocated people cope with their bleak existence. (12) Addiction often becomes the central focus of a person's life and can fill the painful void associated with an absence of belonging. Addictive behaviour serves an adaptive function, but it does so with substantial harm to the individual. It is not the kind of adaptation that people generally want for themselves or that their societies want for them. Yet in a strange but real way, addiction provides people with a sense of belonging, identity, meaning, and purpose despite the associated guilt, remorse and medical consequences. Without their addictions, many people would have terrifyingly little reason to live and risk falling into incapacitating depression or suicide. Addicts overcome the emptiness of their existence by staying very busy chasing their high. They build a life around their habit.

The adaptive function of addiction is often hidden. Many addicted people deny that they live in a state of dislocation, because they feel ashamed of their inability to find a secure, whole and meaningful life, a sense of who they are, some values they can believe in, a place they can call their own, or a reason to get up in the morning. They may deny their dislocation because it feels like an unbearable personal failure and they may be unaware of the adaptive function of their addiction. This conceptualization of addiction aptly applies to the lives of so many of the homeless addicts we see at Siloam.

Characterizing addiction as a response to negative social forces will influence how we respond to it. It steers us away from a "war on drugs" approach—criminalizing a person's maladaptive response to suffering—and points us to the goal of establishing addicted people in a welcoming community that allows them to find healthy meaning and purpose for their lives. Initiatives like 'restoring communities', 'recovery houses' and 'support groups' fit within this model.

We see many patients at the Mission desperate to get clean and sober. Providing medical clearance for a patient who wants to enter an alcohol and drug rehabilitation program is one of the daily jobs at the homeless shelter clinic. The candidates come to the clinic at the end of their rope. They are tired, in trouble, alone, and begging for help. It is tragic how many people fail in their attempts at abstinence, back on the bottle, back in conflict, and back in the clinic, praying that this time it will be different. This time they will succeed. One patient I saw embodied the fact that alcohol can literally destroy a person. It can leave you tortured by real and imaginary enemies. There are some things you see in a homeless shelter medical clinic that you just don't see anywhere else. This case still makes my skin crawl.

I was working a Friday morning shift at the Mission, when my next patient literally burst into the examining room. He was a disheveled Caucasian male in his mid-fifties who looked twenty years older. He was agitated, and expletives filled the air. He was scratching his skin furiously, with excoriated tracks up and down his arms. He was mad about the beds at this "f---ing" Mission, and furious that he had contracted bed bugs here. He was so "f---ing" itchy that he wanted me to cut his skin off! He demanded treatment immediately, or he was going to the media and heads were going to roll. His language was much more colorful than that rendered here. It became apparent in a matter of minutes that he was confused and I wondered if he was delusional. The potential for bed bugs is taken very seriously by the Mission, so I had them check to see where he was sleeping. The clinic staff investigated the matter and told me he had never slept at Siloam. His medical chart was relatively thin, with a few comments about abusive behavior and poor conduct interspersed amongst notes about suspected alcoholism.

We learned the man had his own room at a Main Street hotel, in the toughest part of our city where the poor eke out a marginalized existence. It seemed he was one of the poor souls whose brains are permanently damaged by alcohol. I wondered whether he might be going through withdrawal. Alcohol withdrawal is a remarkably dangerous condition, with a host of dangerous manifestations. A broad range of syndromes can develop, ranging from agitation to seizures and delirium, where a patient develops hallucinations and delusions. A potential symptom is *formication*, where the patient's skin feels like it is crawling with insects. I wondered whether my angry patient was formicating, when the real cause became abundantly clear.

I went to check the man's vital signs to determine if he was in alcohol withdrawal, when I saw the problem. As I put the blood pressure cuff on his arm, I saw that his skin literally *was* crawling. I could see lice crawling on his head, through his beard and on his arms. They were scattered all over his clothes. I instantly felt my own skin crawl, and it became difficult to stay in the same room as the man. I had to push through my own phobia of insects to remain with him. Running out of an examination room screaming is very bad form.

It was difficult to get any reliable medical history from the patient, as he was so agitated with his "f---ing" itch. I didn't blame him. I started to itch everywhere, convinced I was being colonized by the parasites. I had never seen such an infestation. I just wanted to get this man treated and out of the clinic.

The Mission has a stockpile of donated medications, and the pesticide needed to kill the lice was in the stockroom. I walked the patient through the necessary steps to apply the lotion to his head and body and gave him an information sheet on the product. He seemed to acknowledge the instructions, the need to wash his bedsheets and clothes, to shave his head and beard and examine all the surfaces in his suite. We wrote all the necessary steps on a discharge form for him. The room he had been examined in had to be fumigated and was "off limits" for the rest of the morning. The last thing the Mission needed was the additional burden of being labelled a breeding ground for lice.

I felt my skin crawl the rest of the morning, sure that some of my patient's lice had migrated to me. I was glad to see the man go, and thankful that we were able to help him. Unfortunately, the reality of his situation required much more than my boy scout routine provided. I didn't know how naïve I was.

I was back at the Mission the following Friday when it seemed like a scene from the film, *Groundhog Day*. Patient no. 9 was the man with the crawling skin and the "f---ing" itch. He began our interaction with the identical series of expletives he had used the week before. It was clear that to him, we had never met. He had no recollection of our visit or my very explicit treatment recommendations. He again blamed his plight on the "f---ing" bedbugs in the "f---ing" mission, and didn't seem to notice the legion of lice crawling all over his body. This time he stated he was sleeping at another facility and threatened to go to the media about their unsanitary conditions. We confirmed that he had not slept there either.

It became clear that our patient probably had alcoholic dementia and was one of the many people not sick enough to be in an institution but not well enough to have a reasonable life on his own. He was able to navigate the streets without a yesterday, and with no real hope for tomorrow. He simply reacted to the torments of the day. Today was a battle against an infestation of lice that was literally covering his body. Today we had to take control of this situation. The larger problem of how to help the man live a life of dignity was one of those systemic issues that didn't really seem to have a solution. A compassionate and comprehensive home for people like this man doesn't seem to exist in our community, or in many others across North America. The homeless mission can seem like a band-aid in the face of a hemorrhage.

We decided that we required public health support, someone to go into this man's hotel room and clean things up, as we feared he would never be free of his problem without such interventions. Simply giving him the lice-killing lotion and educational materials, as I had done so earnestly the week before, was an exercise in futility.

The public health representatives called back and asked if we were sure the client had lice, and not bedbugs. I told them I could see the lice clearly, on his head and on his body and clothes. They responded that I was mistaken, that head lice and body lice do not occur simultaneously, and that he probably had bedbug bites. Then they asked if I had considered scabies. I assured them that the lice were clearly visible, and suggested they come down to the Mission and verify the problem for themselves. To my amazement, two public health workers arrived at the Mission about a half hour later. Although my memory may be colored by what felt like a condescending attitude, I see them dressed in pantsuits with clipboards in hand and muttering "tsk, tsk" convinced they were wasting their time. I escorted them into the examining room and introduced them to our patient. In a matter of seconds, they were running out of the room wriggling and squirming. Bad form indeed. I was so glad it was them running out of the room and not me.

They acknowledged the presence of both head and body lice and agreed to send a fumigation team into his hotel room. We agreed to shave the patient's head and beard and provide him with a new set of clothes, followed by a trip to a local government clinic for the application of the medication to kill the lice left on his body. People gave him a wide berth as he finally headed out of the clinic. He seemed gratified that we were finally dealing with the "bedbugs".

I saw the man again about a month later, at first not recognizing him with his freshly shaven head and face. The excoriations on his arms were healing, and he seemed to be free of the lice. But it was now patently clear that he had alcoholic dementia, as we had been able to get some medical information from the detox unit at the hospital. His prospects for the future were poor. The man was ranting about new complaints, using the same expletives to inform me of his troubles. I developed a compulsive itch just seeing him.

The burden of this man's world seemed insurmountable. We may have achieved a small victory ridding him of the lice, but the battle of his alcohol addiction still lay ahead. You will not see images of this man in a beer commercial. I haven't seen him since, but he left a permanent impression in my mind. While his condition may have been self-inflicted, who knows what pain he was trying to forget, what hell he was trying to numb with the booze. I suspect his thirst was not for alcohol, but for elusive things like love, forgiveness, acceptance and relief. I'm sure he had never heard of the concepts of dislocation and social fragmentation, but I'm equally sure he experienced them.

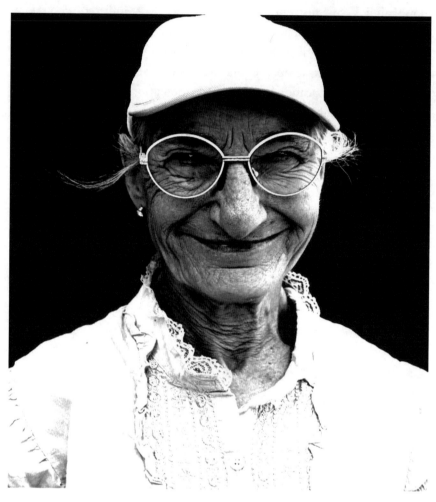

This photograph is taken with permission from Leah Denbok's work, *Nowhere to Call Home. Photographs and Stories of the Homeless. Volume One* or her website. It is not an image of any character referred to in this book. To see more of Leah's photography, visit ldenbokphotography.com.

LESSON 4: You may see more smiles at a homeless shelter than at a country club.

"It is one of the most beautiful compensations of life, that no man can sincerely try to help another without helping himself."
—Ralph Waldo Emerson

I've often marveled at the reaction from people on the street when someone responds positively to a request for money. The most frequent reply is, "God bless you." God bless *me*? I'm the one with the money and the ability to give, and you're living on the street, and you want God to bless *me*? I always found this such a paradox. One of the lessons I have learned from working at the homeless shelter is that, when I try to serve another person with kindness, they end up giving me much more than I give them. One of the treasures the homeless share with me most is their joy in the midst of sorrow.

People living on the street endure difficulties that most of us can't imagine. I'm often amazed at the joy that many of them manifest despite their circumstances. As a Canadian doctor, I am well paid and, as a consequence, I have had the privilege of being to some amazing places. I remember walking in the Whistler Village on a guys' ski trip to British Columbia and coining the phrase, "Joyless in Paradise." I noticed so many presumably affluent people walking around but it seemed that nobody was smiling. The buddy I was with observed the same phenomenon and it became a recurring theme of our time there: bounty in one's bank account does not guarantee gratitude or joy in one's spirit. I contrast this with the Mission where joy and laughter are found, often in abundance. The positive outlook I see in the workers is one thing, and perhaps could be explained away, but the joy in some of the homeless people is mystifying and inspiring. These strong and resilient people can manage to smile in what is anything but paradise.

Eva was an example of this joy in difficult circumstances. She was my last patient of the morning. In fact, we had a hard time finding her as she had disappeared from the waiting room. We eventually found Eva sipping coffee in the common room. I encountered a 67-year old Indigenous woman, her face deeply lined from a life on the street. Slight and feisty, she weighed less than 100 pounds but was an enormous presence in the room. Eva had her left arm in a partial cast and held it at her side in a sling. She said that her broken arm had become painful overnight and she was worried something had happened to it. She had fractured it two weeks earlier but could not recall which bones had been broken. She had undergone an open reduction and internal fixation with a titanium plate used to stabilize her fracture. We attempted to get further information from the large hospital in our catchment area but couldn't make contact with their medical records department. We had only one course of action - to remove her cast and inspect her arm.

The cast was already cut in two, often done to allow the swelling in an injured extremity to wax and wane. We cut the gauze holding the halves together and opened up the cast. Underneath was an angry incision with crusted blood pulling at steri-strips. A second wound was sutured together, with the stitches buried deep in the crusty scab. The arm was swollen but did not appear infected. I removed the strips holding the first wound together and that seemed to ease some of the tension in the skin and, with it, the pain Eva was experiencing. I could feel a plate beneath her skin and I asked her if she had any definite follow-up plans at the hospital. She did not want to talk about the hospital and did not want to return there.

Eva was thankful that her pain had diminished by simple removal of the steri-strips but was worried when I told her it was time to remove the sutures from her arm. They were disappearing into the maturing scab and beginning to look inflamed. Eva started to cry when I suggested she lie down so I could remove the sutures. She was so tiny and anxious I was concerned she might faint, as suture removal can be painful when the stitches have been swallowed up by the healing process. Her tears ran down over her temples and dripped onto on the examining table. I tried to reassure her that this would not be a major ordeal but she wept at the prospect of more suffering. I imagined there had been much suffering in her past, with many tragedies contributing to the lines etched on her face.

I took the first stitch out. It was buried by several millimeters of mature scab which made it difficult to locate the loop of suture material that has to be cut to allow removal of the entire stitch. I could feel Eva's tension and hoped I wasn't hurting her. When I told her that the first of the sutures had been removed, she was delighted to realize that there had been no pain at all. She told me that she was praying for me. We still had a long way to go, since there were many stitches, all encased in exuberant scab, so I was thankful for the supernatural support. Every time I removed a stitch without pain, she became more thankful, reminding me that her prayers were being answered. Removing sutures is not high on the list of medical competencies, so to be commended effusively for a basic procedure was a first for me. I had never been praised for removing sutures before. Ten stitches were removed, ten prayers were answered and ten commendations were given by my charming little patient.

Eva sat up after we had finished cleaning the dried blood from her forearm. She was delighted at how good her arm felt, and how much better it looked when we cleaned the area. I placed a dry dressing over her wound and she was so thankful for the whole experience. It was at this point that I started to do a little praying of my own. Eva was unaware that I might still have to send her back to the hospital. The Mission clinic does not carry casting material and she required further immobilization of the fracture.

Patrons at Siloam are wary of going to the neighboring tertiary care hospital. The infamous case of a homeless Indigenous person who waited over 30 hours in its triage area and died from septic shock continues to stain its reputation. Mr. Sinclair was a double above-knee amputee who had a urinary catheter in place. He had developed a urinary tract infection and been sent in to the hospital for a catheter change. He presented himself to the triage desk, was registered, and then waited for over a day before someone realized he had died in his wheelchair. It was determined that Mr. Sinclair died of septic shock, a condition that could have been prevented by the simple change of his catheter and antibiotics. The case attracted nation-wide attention and prompted a provincial inquiry into his death. Concerns over emergency room workload, the triage process and systemic racism came to the fore. I was hopeful that we would not require the resources of the hospital for Eva.

Siloam is fortunate to have an assortment of donated orthopedic supplies and splints in its storage area, but to find a suitable rigid splint that would fit Eva's tiny left wrist seemed a tall order. I said a little prayer myself and went to look at our inventory. Much to my amazement, we had exactly one upper extremity splint remaining. It was perfect. Brand new, in the box, left arm, exact length to cover 2/3 of her forearm and removable with velcro straps to facilitate dressing changes. I was thankful. I took the splint back to Eva, and she was ecstatic. It was like I had given her jewelry on Christmas morning. She showed off the splint in the most adorable way, doing the cutest impression of a runway model. She thanked the clinic staff profusely. She danced a little jig with me in her exuberance. She called our clinic assistant into the examination room to show her the new splint and told the woman about her answers to prayer. She then gave me a big hug, full of joy and genuine affection. Her face beamed with the most beautiful smile, exquisitely framed by the lines on her face. I couldn't stop smiling either.

The joy of this single interaction with a patient was extraordinary. No ski resort, golf club, night at the bar, ball game or Broadway show could rival the feeling that Little Eva gave me at a homeless shelter in the toughest part of our town on a cold winter morning. A simple encounter with a homeless person had warmed my heart. Eva taught me that you just may see more smiles at a homeless shelter than a country club.

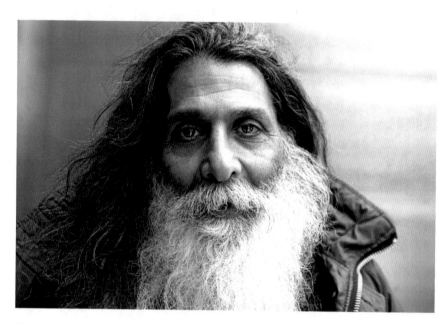

This photograph is taken with permission from Leah Denbok's work, *Nowhere to Call Home. Photographs and Stories of the Homeless. Volume One* or her website. It is not an image of any character referred to in this book. To see more of Leah's photography, visit ldenbokphotography.com.

LESSON 5: Love is corrupted by pride and fear. Pride causes us to love ourselves more than our neighbor, fear makes our neighbors enemies.

God sends no one away empty except those that are full of themselves.
—*D.L. Moody*

Pride is concerned with who is right. Humility is concerned with what is right.
—*Ezra Benson*

Too many of us are not living our dreams because we are living our fears.
—*Les Brown*

After a Christmas party with some family friends, I learned I am a "humble bragger." My daughter, Abby, is a strong young woman, fiercely committed to important causes. She is an ardent feminist, a vegetarian and a protector of the environment. At the party, I talked a lot about my volunteer work at Siloam. When we got home, I felt good about the evening, having made some new friends. I must admit, I felt some pride that the people at the party had seemed impressed by my service at the Mission. Sadly, pride comes before destruction. (13) Abby told me that I should "watch the humble bragging." She rightly observed that I had been trying to impress people with my work for the homeless. I was disappointed in myself when Abby shared this with me because I knew it was true. My pride had been evident and then, paradoxically, I felt fear. I was afraid of what the people at the party would think of me. Had I sounded like a bragger to them? Had arrogance and hubris tainted their perception of me? Would they conclude that my motivation to work at the shelter was just a form of virtue-signaling? People hate a bragger. I thought I had learned this lesson the summer before, with a patient I had treated at the Mission. The story of Pop was emblematic of our tendency to allow pride, insecurity, and anxiety to corrupt our lives.

Pop's story began with a bearded man slumped over in the waiting room of the Mission clinic. We escorted him slowly back to the examination room. He had normal vital signs but was basically catatonic. The nurse administrator had told me that Pop was probably from Sri Lanka and likely had a history of schizoaffective disorder, a common ailment of those living on the street. Schizoaffective disorder is a chronic but treatable psychiatric condition, characterized by periods of normal function punctuated by episodes of depression or mania. The patients may manifest psychosis, where individuals lose touch with reality and can experience hallucinations or delusions. Pop had apparently been off his medication for months, was non-communicative and wanted to sleep all the time. He was not unpleasant but simply had no desire or ability to interact with people or his surroundings. How did he get to the Mission? What condition was he suffering from? What brought him to a homeless shelter in Winnipeg?

Through some excellent detective work by the clinic staff, it was discovered that Pop had been on a potent anti-psychotic drug known as Zyprexa when he lived in another Canadian city. We tried several times to confirm this with him, but Pop was unable to talk to us, lost in his own silent and isolated world. He had allowed us to do basic blood tests and a physical examination, and we found no other medical problem to account for his behavior. We decided that we would trust the results of our investigative work and asked Pop if we could prescribe him Zyprexa. He seemed agreeable, but all answers were just a single word. Pop, are you in pain? No. Do you have any medical problems? No. Have you been on Zyprexa before? Yes. Did it help you? Yes. Would you be willing to go back on this? Yes. Do you have any allergies? No. So, we proceeded. We started Pop on the Zyprexa, funded by the Mission, and waited to see if it would help.

I was back at the clinic the subsequent Friday morning, and the transformation in Pop was near miraculous. He was my first patient of the day and I was astounded by how animated he was. He had a brilliant smile and seemed to be getting along famously with everyone. He was articulate and intelligent. From then on, Pop became one of our favorite clients. He was kind, considerate and charming. He had an easy laugh and was always smiling. Over time, we started to fill in the blanks about the journey that had brought Pop to Winnipeg. He had enjoyed a successful life as an engineer after moving from Sri Lanka to the United States, but that was cut short by his mental illness. He had bounced around Canada, trying to find the next chapter in his life.

People with bipolar schizoaffective disorder often feel trapped on their medication. They feel their creativity and zest for life are impaired by the sedating effects of the drugs. This frequently prompts the patient to go off their medication and, for a brief interlude, they feel *themselves* again. In time, though, the good feeling off of medication can be replaced by tangential thoughts, urges of hyper-sexuality or fiscal extravagance, or the opposite, a withdrawn and depressed state. This conundrum plagues the treatment of many mental health patients.

Back on his medication, Pop seemed great. He was the model of equanimity. His communication tended to be grandiose, his language peppered with hyperbole. The food at the Mission was the "best ever," his day "sensational." He told me he could sense that I was a "special person", which I considered to represent significant clarity of thought. Pop did so well on his Zyprexa that he began to volunteer around the Mission. In fact, he became one of Siloam's spokespeople, his smiling face featured on brochures and posters advertising the Mission's services. This man was an example of the joy people can experience in very difficult circumstances. Pop didn't complain about living in a homeless Mission. He was focused on helping others and he seemed content, grateful and at peace.

One day that summer, I was driving with a friend and I saw Pop's picture on the back of a bus in a fundraising ad. I said to my friend "Hey, there's *my patient,* Pop! I look after him at Siloam." I told my friend all about Pop to impress him with my community service. It was a humble brag, perhaps minus the humble. I let my pride get the best of me. My comments were even more inappropriate since I hadn't been at the Mission clinic for several months. I had done nothing to help Pop in quite some time.

The next time I walked into Siloam, I learned Pop was dead. He had developed a particularly aggressive form of cancer and passed away within weeks of his diagnosis. This devastated the Mission staff, as they were very fond of him. It was hard on me as well. I had enjoyed my relationship with this unique fellow. I hate to admit it, but I also worried that my friend would learn that Pop was dead. Some doctor I was. Pride again gave way to fear, insecurity and anxiety.

Practitioners of mindfulness talk about the importance of living in the moment. This concept encourages people to stop letting regrets about the past or worries about the future taint our experience of the present. Similar teachings exist in many faith traditions and most of us can relate to their truth. A related concept is demonstrated by my experience with Pop. I find I often let the emotions of pride and fear rob me of accurate self-perception and the potential for joy in the present. For me, pride and fear are two sides of a well-worn coin.

I am not alone with this fear problem. Anxiety and insecurity are remarkably common, with 15% of people having a bona fide anxiety disorder. Worry and fear seem to color so much of our thought life. The Biblical axiom to "be anxious for nothing" seems an elusive goal. (14) People are afraid of death and dying, illness, terrorism, environmental catastrophe, climate change, and global epidemics. We worry about our financial future, job security, our children and other relationships, aging and infirmity. In addition to the dire health consequences these emotions inflict on people, fear, anxiety and insecurity crowd out thoughts of gratitude, contentment and concerns for the welfare of others. Fear exacts a heavy toll on our health, wellness and enjoyment of life.

Pride can be a more difficult mindset to recognize in ourselves. The alienating effect of pride is easy to spot around boasting and arrogance, but its pervasive nature goes beyond those obvious manifestations. Pride is woven into so many of the qualities that define success in our culture – confidence, the drive to excel, the besting of all competitors in the field – to the point where it is often characterized as a strength and a virtue. That certainly is not its scriptural characterization. The Old Testament says rather that "pride is an abomination." (15)

As I reflect on my relationship with Pop, I realize I was privileged to have known him and to have witnessed his journey back to reality. He demonstrated the importance of having gratitude for the smallest of blessings. He did not seem to be living in fear or corrupted by pride. Pop taught me that many of my fears are actually borne out of my pride. How do I look to others?—a question prompted by pride and culminating in fear. Pop (and my daughter) taught me a lesson I need to learn over and over again: that pride and fear can live side by side in my spirit, and both corrupt my expression of who I really am. Pride causes me to love myself more than others, and fear makes my neighbors enemies. Wisdom from the homeless.

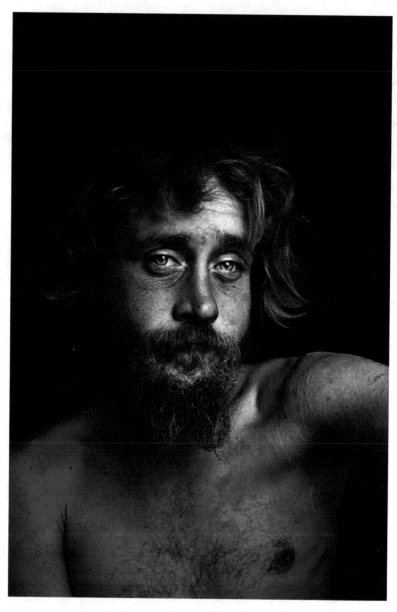

This photograph is taken with permission from Leah Denbok's work, *Nowhere to Call Home. Photographs and Stories of the Homeless. Volume One* or her website. It is not an image of any character referred to in this book. To see more of Leah's photography, visit ldenbokphotography.com.

LESSON 6: I am the prodigal son every time I search for unconditional love where it cannot be found.

—Henri Nouwen

The difference between mercy and grace? Mercy gave the prodigal son a second chance. Grace gave him a feast.
—Max Lucado

He was a quiet man. The entrance complaint on the electronic medical record was simply "Needs burn cream." I thought this would be a simple prescription for a commonly-used burn antibiotic or perhaps a dressing change. The homeless patients I see at Siloam often have significant dermatological problems requiring regular dressings and wound care. Burns, infected blisters from poorly fitting shoes, skin breakdown from neglected leg edema and varicose veins are all very common. This man would require much more than a simple dressing.

Jadon was a memorable fellow. He was clad in traditional gang banger attire. Black hoodie, baggy black sweats, and a black toque overflowing with an untamed mop of blond hair which framed his piercing blue eyes. He was a Caucasian man in his early twenties with a beard that seemed to be six inches long and equally untamed. He had what the medical community describes as a Marfanoid appearance: remarkably tall, probably 6'6", slender, with extremely long limbs. He had a steely glare while sitting in the waiting room, but there was something vulnerable about him. I asked him how I could help him and he said in a matter-of-fact way, "I need some burn cream." A simple request. I asked him to show me his burn and he slowly rose from his chair and began to remove his hoody. I was speechless when I saw his torso. He had widespread partial and full-thickness burns over his entire chest and abdomen. A red mass of angry scale and healing skin grafts gave the impression of a badly traumatized reptile. Some of the areas were infected with mild cellulitis. The skin was thick, raw and in places, bleeding, leaving multiple areas of blood on the inside of his hoody.

I tried to conceal my reaction but I was dumbstruck by the worst burn I had ever seen. How did this happen? Jadon reluctantly told me he was the victim of attempted murder. Some bad actors had tried to kill him by trapping him in a burning building. He clearly didn't want to go into the specifics, just wanting some attention to his troubled skin. I didn't push for any more information but was so curious to hear his story; I hadn't met many people who had survived an ordeal in a homicidal inferno. He mumbled that he was lucky to be alive.

Jadon told me that a nurse had really helped him by applying derma-base to the burns. This is a lubricating, soothing commercial cream that the Mission carries in its medicine cupboard. It would be easy to do this for him.

I got the dermabase from the cupboard and had Jadon lie down. His long frame did not fit on the examination plinth and he had to bend his knees and hips to get comfortable. His skin was raw and fragile, yet thick and rough, bleeding easily when too much force was applied. As a consequence, gentle manual pressure had to be used. The whole scene was so incongruous. Me, the doc from the suburbs, massaging medicinal cream on the entire abdomen and chest of a victim of homicidal violence. I didn't want to tell Jadon that I felt something spiritual in this act. This man was encased in a thick husk of reptilian skin, pain etched on his face. But I could see his jaw relax as the cream brought some relief. He trusted me, and I wanted to ease his pain.

We began to chat, and I discovered that he was the same age as my son. Two young men on very different paths. My son, safe and sound and now attending medical school, and Jadon, recovering from life threatening burns he sustained in a brutal attempt on his life. We joked a little and Jadon started to open up. His life had been hijacked by drug deals and substance abuse. The party life hadn't provided the acceptance he was looking for. It sounded as though he had known little of love, encouragement or affirmation in his whole life. His family had disintegrated and I wondered if this was one of the things he was running from. I commented on how tough he must be to tolerate his painful condition in such a stoic manner. He smirked, and I suspected that that had been his trademark on the street.

Jadon had some burns that required debridement - removal of dead skin using forceps and scissors – followed by special dressings with antibiotic cream and non-adhering gauze. The whole process probably took half an hour. As we dealt with his burns, I began to feel a connection with the young man. His demeanor softened and he actually smiled when I encouraged him to book his next *spa* treatment. I told him I didn't do nails, bikini waxing or pedicures. He laughed and left.

I saw Jadon a week later. He wanted another "treatment", and I was pleased to provide it. The same routine was done with inspection for infection, debridement of dead skin, slow massage of cream into the thickened epidermis, and dressing of infected burns. We talked most of the time. Near the end of his visit, I asked him if he had any plans for his future. He told me that he was still facing criminal charges and could be going back to the penitentiary. This young man, permanently scarred, frightened and homeless, might be headed back to jail. I asked when he would learn of his sentence, and he told me that he expected to know the week before Christmas. I had a clinic at Siloam on the 24th of December and told him I would pray for him. He nodded and left.

When I got to my shift on the 24th, Jadon was not on the day's appointment list. I had looked forward to seeing him, hoping he would have some good news to share. As I wound down the clinic that day, I told the story of my interaction with Jadon to the clinic triage person. I voiced my disappointment that I hadn't got to see him one last time. She told me that he had in fact been by the clinic and asked to see me, but she thought I was too busy and told him that a nurse could help him the following day.

She thought she was cutting me a break, unaware of the legal limbo that Jadon was in. I was surprised how disappointed I felt that I wouldn't see Jadon again.

The parable of the prodigal son is one of my favorite stories. (16) The image of the Father waiting for his son to return after his time of wild living speaks volumes about God. The Father runs out to meet his repentant son and showers love on him. Repentance dismissed the need for judgment and amazing grace is offered. The son has a second chance at life with his family. There was no finger wagging, no I told you so. Guilt and shame are not discussed. There is an emotional reunion, characterized by an embrace between Father and son. I have felt that embrace. I wished that Jadon could feel it as well. I have no idea what has happened to him. I simply have to keep praying.

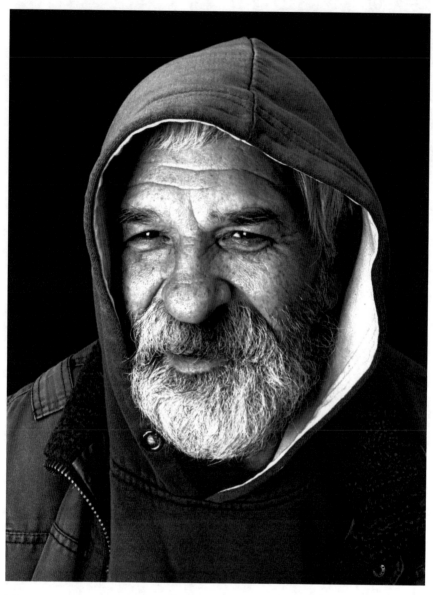

This photograph is taken with permission from Leah Denbok's work, *Nowhere to Call Home. Photographs and Stories of the Homeless. Volume One* or her website. It is not an image of any character referred to in this book. To see more of Leah's photography, visit ldenbokphotography.com.

LESSON 7: You could be the next Good Samaritan.

No act of kindness, however small, is ever wasted.
—Aesop

I volunteer in the Mission clinic twice a month. I often wonder if that's enough. Should I bother to go if I can't make a more substantial investment of time? Is my service just a token, not representative of real commitment? Does it make any difference? These are questions that float through my subconsciousness from time to time. There are only a handful of docs who work at the Mission, so it does seem to be necessary. One Friday I was caught off-guard by the comments of one of my patients, and he convinced me that *no act of kindness is ever wasted*.

Near the end of my shift, I noticed a familiar face who had been waiting most of the morning to see me. Dave was a friendly guy who remembered my name and needed some help. I had seen him at the Mission clinic many times over the years. Siloam encourages people to find more consistent medical care than what can be provided by the volunteers who serve sporadically at the Mission. There are some excellent government-funded clinics in the neighborhood, with substantial staff and resources to serve the core area population. Still, many people prefer to come to the Mission clinic and have been doing so for years.

Dave had hurt his shoulder working on a pipeline and was having trouble continuing with his job. While I sometimes feel out of my league dealing with the array of medical problems that can afflict those on the street, shoulders are something I know. My real job is sports medicine, and I felt like saying to Dave: *Finally!* A problem I'm competent to deal with.

Dave was worried he had torn his rotator cuff and that it would jeopardize his high-paying employment. I gave Dave a thorough evaluation and after my assessment, I could reassure him that his cuff wasn't torn. He had a common problem that could be rehabilitated. He was thankful that he would be able to keep working. We chatted about his job and his sense of optimism for his future. Dave was on the path back to self-sufficiency and was hoping to have a place of his own in the near future. He was one of Siloam's success stories, moving from homelessness and poverty to a well-paying job, dignity and self-respect.

I began discussing some exercises he could do at home and told him he should follow up with his "family doctor." What he said in response put many things into perspective for me. He said "*This* is my home and *you* are my doctor." I was taken aback by his perception of our relationship and his fondness for the Mission. He wasn't homeless, he had a loving home! He had a doctor and I was him. It was actually gratifying to hear Dave's perspective.

It's easy to feel that periodic volunteering at the Mission doesn't make any difference in the big picture. I felt that my episodic attendances at Siloam wouldn't count much in the lives of those I encountered there. Admittedly, my deepest relationships are grounded by years of common experience. But I have also been changed by people I have known fleetingly. I can remember chance encounters with people from all walks of life who have treated me with kindness and respect. I am the sum of all these encounters. Likewise, my interactions with others, however brief, make a contribution to who they become.

Dave helped me understand that no act of kindness, however small, is ever wasted. The world has celebrated the action of the Good Samaritan for 2000 years. (17) This parable communicates so many important truths. Jesus told the story as an answer to a hostile question about loving our neighbor. Who are our neighbors? Are they people like us? From our own community or family? White guys from the suburbs? Jesus taught that our neighbors encompass all people whose lives intersect with ours, regardless of their class, religion, sexuality, ethnicity or circumstances. In fact, He emphasized that our neighbors - those people we are to love - are those we would characterize as enemies. Every single person I rub shoulders with, anywhere I go, is my neighbor.

We only know of the Samaritan's one act of kindness to a person in need, yet he is the world's icon of selfless service across the ethnic divide. Dave reminded me that one act can alter the trajectory of a person's life. And who knows, you may be the next Good Samaritan, the person who showed us what it means to truly "Love your neighbor as you love yourself." (17)

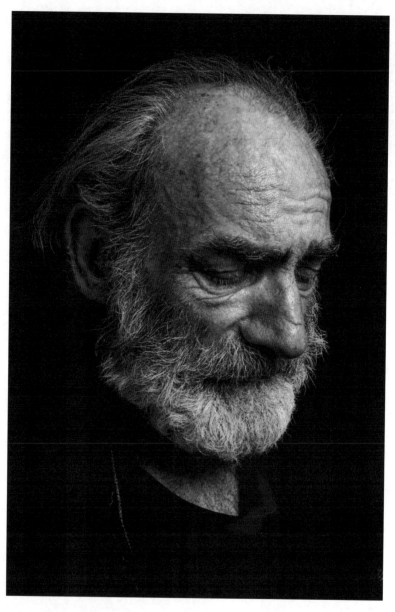

This photograph is taken with permission from Leah Denbok's work, *Nowhere to Call Home. Photographs and Stories of the Homeless. Volume One* or her website. It is not an image of any character referred to in this book. To see more of Leah's photography, visit ldenbokphotography.com.

LESSON 8: Holding a grudge doesn't make you strong, it makes you bitter. Forgiving someone doesn't make you weak, it sets you free.

—DaveWillis.org

Never look down on somebody unless you're helping him up.
—Jesse Jackson

There is an amazing cast of characters at the Mission. Many of them are paradoxically joyful and love to share a laugh. One elderly man stands out in my mind—probably 70 years old, tall, brash, boisterous and loud, with a thick Scottish accent. He was not your average grandpa figure. He had purple hair. His larger-than-life persona colored our entire visit. I can't recall why he wanted medical help, but he definitely wanted to engage in robust banter. My surname, "Craton", has distinctly Scottish roots. A *craton* is the "stable interior portion of a continent characteristically composed of ancient crystalline basement rock" – in short, a rock outcropping. My purple-haired patient must have known this obscure fact. He asked me to spell my name and, once he confirmed his suspicion, christened me "Rocky." Every part of our conversation was punctuated with the epithet. "Thanks for your help, Rocky", he giggled, as he left the examination room. He tried to get the staff to call me Rocky for the rest of the day.

The next patient was an old man who seemed vaguely familiar. He also looked 70, used a cane and ambulated slowly. His forward-flexed posture indicated chronic spinal problems. I checked the name on the day sheet and immediately recognized it. The name had been etched in my mind since adolescence. Lance had not aged well. The athleticism of his youth was gone. His story was a sad one.

I remember Lance as being the best player on our Junior High basketball team. He matured early and was probably 5'10" by the time he was 13. Lance was very athletic and very muscular, a man among boys. I recall a game when Lance scored all of our points and doubled the output of the other team. It seemed as though every time Lance touched the ball he scored, since his prepubescent competitors - mere mortals – couldn't stop him. Those moments are firmly fixed in my memory because I was one of his envious prepubescent teammates. Lance could do things that the rest of us couldn't, and most of us didn't see ourselves ever navigating puberty and the changes that would hopefully ensue.

Lance also had a mean streak. At 13, I was a terrible basketball player. Lance regularly mocked me and we actually came to blows after a game where my ineptitude probably caused our team to lose. I did not fare well in the brief altercation. At school, Lance would throw a punch at me whenever our paths crossed and he made sure that all the girls heard his disparaging comments about me. This humiliation haunted my early adolescence and still reminds me of the vulnerability of youth. The bullying persisted from Grade 7 to Grade 10. Suffice it to say I came to have negative feelings about Lance.

Over the summer between Grade 10 and 11, something amazing happened. I hit puberty. I grew almost 6 inches and gained close to fifty pounds. I remember coming back to school and thinking that everyone had shrunk over the summer. Lance was looking for me to mete out his usual punishment and was taken aback to see my transformation. I probably outweighed him by those fifty pounds. He took a swing at me but I dodged it, put him in a wrestling hold and threw him to the ground. I knelt on his chest and said "Lance, this is over." I never heard another word from him. But I must confess that my feelings of fear and animosity towards Lance remained vivid in my mind.

Later in high school, Lance sustained a serious injury while bumper shining. For those who don't live where the streets are icy, bumper shining is the sport of grabbing hold of the fender of a slowly-moving vehicle, squatting down and basically skiing behind the car. Most of us engaged in this risky sport in our adolescence. While bumper shining, Lance had slipped under the vehicle and had sustained serious orthopedic injuries. Those injuries changed his future and initiated his long downhill journey to the homeless shelter medical clinic.

During our visit in the clinic, Lance seemed bright and articulate. He didn't recognize me at first, as we hadn't seen each other since high school. He was quite shocked when I reminded him that we had been teammates over forty years ago. Lance and I didn't talk about the five years of bullying. We talked about his back pain and his current life, trying to re-establish himself. Lance told me that the accident had left him with chronic pain, another burden commonly faced by the homeless. Despite his problems, he had started a successful business and, at one point, had been a wealthy man. But the opioids he had been using to treat his pain had got the best of him.

Opioids have become one of the predominant problems in North American culture. These analgesics are effective for short term pain relief and palliative care. However, through aggressive and dishonest marketing techniques, they became a staple in the treatment of chronic, benign, musculoskeletal pain syndromes. Use of these medications rapidly leads to tolerance, a situation where the dose has to be increased to obtain the same degree of pain relief. They also lead to dependence, where any decrease in dosage leads to unpleasant withdrawal phenomena. The other lesser-known consequence of this class of drugs is opioid-induced hyperalgesia. This is the effect by which these drugs actually reset the nervous system to make it more sensitive to pain impulses. In essence, they decrease your pain threshold. The same stimulus produces more pain for the sufferer, the neurological condition known as hyperalgesia. Other complications include significant problems with dentition and abnormal hormone function. An unprecedented number of deaths from overdose and respiratory depression has become the most destructive complication of this epidemic.

While the medical literature does not indicate that these drugs are effective for long-term pain management, opioids are powerfully addictive, and so patient demand for them is quite high. Ironically, these medications are insured – in other words, paid for by our government—but pain treatments by physiotherapists, massage therapists and chiropractors are not. The "opioid crisis" has ultimately lead to the fentanyl epidemic, leaving hundreds of addicts dying across North America every month. In 2016, roughly 50,000 Americans died from opioids. More people are killed by opioids than the number who died of HIV at the peak of that epidemic. In Canada and the United States, these drugs kill more people than car crashes and gun violence combined. Sadly, the abuse of opioids and the painful burden they create are a common thread among the patients described on these pages.

Despite these significant adverse consequences, opioids are everywhere, particularly on the street. I regularly tell patients at the Mission clinic that we do not prescribe opioids, for fear of diversion and the dire consequences of these drugs in the homeless world. Diversion is the practice where a patient is prescribed an opioid and it finds its way into the hands of someone other than the patient. It is an enormous problem. After telling one man at the clinic that I would not be willing to prescribe him opioids, he said he understood and simply asked me which drug I would recommend for his chronic back pain, the consequence of an industrial accident. I asked him why he wanted to know. He told me that he was just going to go out on the street and get what I recommended, because all the opioids were available for easy purchase just outside our door. He told me that a Fentanyl patch would sell for close to $250. A crazy world indeed.

Lance had begun using opioids early in his life. As with most patients, there had been a honeymoon period where the analgesics seemed to work, making him feel better. However, the unholy triad of dependence, tolerance and opioid-induced hyperalgesia quickly ambushed him. In the typical case, the opioid requirement escalates and the person starts using "non-prescription opioids", which is usually code for heroin. At that point, the person often descends into the abyss of opioid addiction. People lose everything, including their businesses. That's what happened to Lance. The once-invincible athlete was visiting a homeless shelter medical clinic, bankrupt and barely able to walk. Lance reminded me of the thin line that separates all of us from a life on the street.

As I talked with Lance and contemplated all that had passed between us those decades ago, and all that had happened to him in the intervening years, I realized that I had not come through the years unscathed either. I had been carrying around a grudge against Lance for his treatment of me; a small festering sore. I held a residual bitterness towards the man, even forty years later. What foolishness to drag around a grievance for half a lifetime. How small-minded not to have given grace for the offenses of a teenager with a host of insecurities of his own. I considered my baggage and I laid it down. I silently forgave him. I felt better immediately.

Lance and I had a good visit. If he remembered terrorizing me, he gave no sign of it. We shared a laugh or two as I outlined some non-opioid suggestions for pain management. I encouraged him to see the Mission physiotherapist. We marveled at how our paths had diverged and then intersected again. In 1972, I would have given anything to be Lance. Now, he was a little old man, desperately in need of help. I was able to forgive him for those long-ago bruises of adolescence. The visit with Lance taught me that holding a grudge doesn't make me strong, it makes me bitter. He taught me that forgiveness doesn't make me weak, it sets me free. I forgave him that day. I felt free indeed.

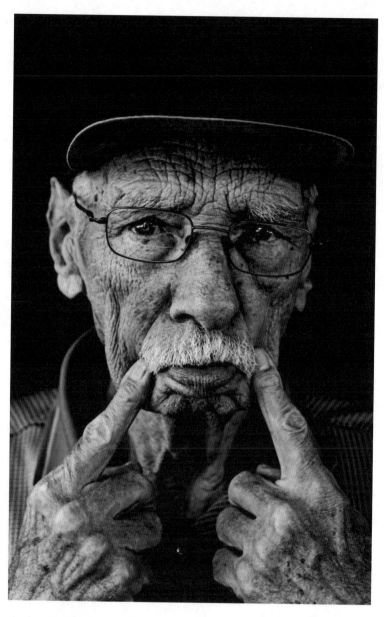

This photograph is taken with permission from Leah Denbok's work, *Nowhere to Call Home. Photographs and Stories of the Homeless. Volume One* or her website. It is not an image of any character referred to in this book. To see more of Leah's photography, visit ldenbokphotography.com.

LESSON 9: Trust is like fine china, formed through fire with intention and care, shattered in a moment.

A lie can travel half way round the world while truth is still putting its shoes on.
—Charles Spurgeon.

Many of the patients we see at the Mission are carrying everything they own with them. Shopping bags and knapsacks full of all kinds of stuff. Clothes, identification, medications, appointment reminders and keepsakes spill out of these portable carry-alls. When I first started at Siloam, I was amazed to find that almost all of the patrons had cell phones. I associated cell phones with affluence, but I was obviously wrong. It has become a necessity of life. One patient who I became quite close to over the years was always carrying around a thick novel. He would regularly recount the plot to me with the elocution of a magistrate. Unfortunately, fiction crept into our relationship and broke the trust I had placed in him.

Jerome was in his early 70's and was in many ways a typical patron of the Mission. He was a black man, with a history of mental health trouble, addiction and incarceration. He was a diminutive character, standing about 5'6" tall and weighing 130 pounds. His silver beard curled wildly and looked to account for half his body weight. Jerome was a bright and engaging historian and I enjoyed our visits, as we discussed the politics of the day alongside his various health problems. He had fascinating stories about his life on the street and in the penitentiary. He related stories where he had outfoxed fellow inmates with his wit and guile, despite his frail stature.

While in the penitentiary, Jerome had taken potent anti-psychotic medications including one called Haldol. This medication, also known as haloperidol, is a powerful tranquilizer, and is often used in emergency rooms to sedate agitated patients. "Vitamin H", as it is affectionately known to ER docs, can transform a raging, threatening and violent patient into a compliant customer. On a prescription basis, it is reserved for psychotic individuals, and was historically used to treat schizophrenia. Newer medications have largely replaced it.

Jerome described himself as having an impulse control disorder. His short fuse had caused him endless trouble, including incarceration on multiple occasions. He hoped that I could prescribe him some medication to keep him calm and avoid violent confrontations with other men on the street. We had a long chat about Siloam's prescription policies. In general, we do not prescribe opioids or benzodiazepines, another class of medication commonly abused on the street. The benzodiazepines are part of the class of medications known as sedative/hypnotics. They were among the first sleeping pills used on a widespread basis and were also given to ameliorate anxiety. While benzodiazepines are still prescribed episodically to treat acute panic attacks, they are seldom used as sedatives or just to help control behavior. They are abused on the street for their sedating effects and are highly addictive. A little-known fact is that the withdrawal effects of benzodiazepines are among the most dangerous of all drugs if patients are addicted. For me to prescribe these medications would be quite a rarity.

Jerome persuaded me otherwise. He seemed to have good insight into his impulse control disorder, acknowledging how much trouble his lack of self-control had caused. He was fed up with the major tranquilizers - Haldol, Seroquel and the like. He was not depressed and felt he didn't need that class of medication. But he was very worried about getting into an altercation and, as a frail older man, knew that such a dust-up might be his last. Psychological counselling is difficult to access for many of the homeless and Jerome said he didn't engage well with therapists. After much discussion of the risks and benefits of benzodiazepines, we agreed to a trial of Ativan, a short-acting anxiolytic medication. We would see how things went for that month and then reassess. Our clinic administrator gave me a sideways glance when she saw I was planning to prescribe Jerome some Ativan, one of the benzodiazepines we usually avoided prescribing. I assured her that I trusted Jerome and went through the logic of using this class of drug in his case - a clear psychiatric past, his impulse control disorder, a reticence to use more potent medication; it all seemed reasonable to me. Furthermore, I pointed out to her, this silver-haired *little old man* would never scam us. She reluctantly agreed.

The plan seemed to work for a few months. Jerome took the appropriate amount of medication and said that he felt better. He was less anxious, sleeping better, and had more patience with the other patrons at the shelter and on the street. During our follow-up visits, it became apparent that Jerome was losing weight. There wasn't much to find on physical examination, and I suggested we start doing some tests to identify the reason for his weight loss. Jerome responded as many street people do: if he was sick, he didn't want to know what was wrong and he was ready to die. This gave me a grudging respect for him, if colored by a hint of melancholy. Did he really have nothing to live for? Against my better judgement, we agreed to just watch and wait, and continue with his benzodiazepines.

A month later, Jerome came in for his medication refill about two weeks earlier than he should have. He related an elaborate tale about a lady friend, staying in his apartment, who had robbed him and beaten him up. He did have a black eye and, for the life of me, I couldn't see this man lying to me. I trusted him and was more than a little shocked that he still had a romantic life. He made some off-hand complaints about his luck with women and we had a bit of a chuckle. I refilled his prescription and sent him on his way. I pestered him to check his weight before he left and he grudgingly cooperated. There had been another two-pound weight loss.

Things began to deteriorate after that, but not with his health. The next visit, Jerome told me he had been mugged on the street and that all his medication had been stolen again. He needed another prescription. He was several weeks early. It seemed so pathetic that this poor old man, living in the toughest part of town, was being assaulted on a regular basis.

He did not want to talk about his assailants, and just asked for his medication. I told him that that was something I wouldn't do for most patients and explained that the medical profession has great concerns about drug diversion. As with opioids, benzodiazepines are very popular on the street, frequently shared, sold or stolen. He assured me that the medications were working well, and that he was the only one taking them. He asserted, rightfully, that he should not be blamed for being mugged. He joked that at least this time he had been beaten up by a man. I relented again.

Jerome returned to the clinic ahead of his scheduled appointment yet again. This time, he told me he was moving to Vancouver and that he was leaving Winnipeg permanently. He said that, if he was dying, he wanted to be able to see the ocean and the mountains one last time. He thanked me for my help over the years and wondered if I could give him a larger supply of the Ativan to ensure he would not run out before finding a doctor in British Columbia. He asked me for a letter confirming that I was prescribing this medication for him, to ease his transition to a new practitioner. I gave him a double prescription of the Ativan and said goodbye to this interesting character. I didn't have many relationships with senior citizens who had spent half of their life in prison and read more books than Kate.

I was very surprised to see Jerome back at the clinic three weeks later. He said his trip to Vancouver had been a disaster. He found the homeless situation there to be dominated by heroin addicts and felt that he was in constant danger. He had been able to panhandle enough money to buy a bus ticket and headed back to Winnipeg. Frankly, I wondered if he had he even gone. Would he lie to me in such a bald-faced manner? Angelika, the clinic administrator, had been very patient with me prescribing medication in contravention of the clinic's rules. I could tell that she was becoming increasingly uncomfortable with this arrangement. I told Jerome that I would not be able to give him any more of the Ativan, and that he would have to develop a relationship with a family physician in the area. My trust was wavering and I could no longer put myself or the Mission in such a difficult position.

In no time at all, Jerome added another twist to his convoluted story. He told me that he was now going to New Brunswick to reconcile with his estranged daughter. He would not be staying in Winnipeg any longer. In his usual articulate fashion, he recounted the trials and tribulations of his relationship with his daughter. He made reference to the fact that he was probably dying and wanting to mend fences with his only child. In his persuasive way, he reminded me of the danger of withdrawing from benzodiazepines, a fact I had shared with him at the beginning of our odyssey. He had tucked this nugget away in his memory when I had tried to discourage him from starting that class of medication in the first place. I found the facts he presented to be compelling, and he was emphatic that he was leaving. Angelika let me decide, and I chose to trust Jerome and give him one final prescription of the benzodiazepines. I gave him some more medication and wished him all the best in his attempts to reconcile with his estranged daughter.

At my next shift, two weeks later, Angelika asked to speak with me before I began seeing patients. Jerome had been caught selling Ativan on the streets in front of the Mission. This frail old man in the middle of the toughest part of our city was a drug dealer, and I had been his stooge. I was embarrassed that I had fallen for his tall tales. I was disappointed that someone would lie so blatantly and without a perceptible scintilla of guilt. I would never prescribe benzodiazepines in that capacity again. I learned the hard lesson that some people will take advantage of a do-gooder and that my naïve desire to see the best in people had made me blind to the realities of life on the street. I learned that institutional policies can reflect the wisdom gained from the mistakes of those who have come before us and ought not to be lightly disregarded. I learned that trust can take a long time to develop but can be destroyed in the blink of an eye.

Angelika tells me she has seen Jerome at the Mission on several occasions since the dust-up. Jerome is apparently clean, sober, and no longer selling drugs on the street. He says that he feels fabulous. He is actually gaining weight. Rumor has it that it was the stress of doing drug deals that caused his weight-loss, not any nefarious medical condition. Angelika has been very gracious, allowing me to learn the lesson of broken trust on my own.

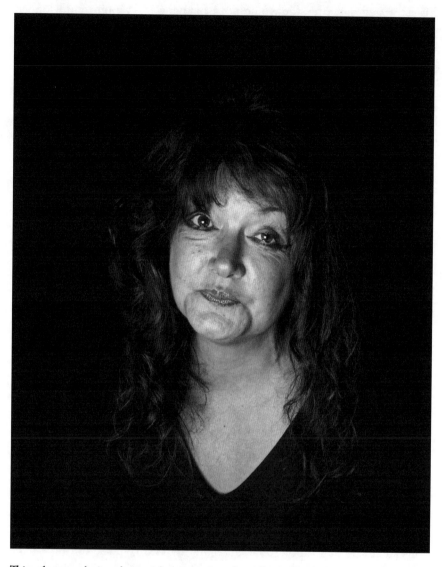

This photograph is taken with permission from Leah Denbok's work, *Nowhere to Call Home. Photographs and Stories of the Homeless. Volume One* or her website. It is not an image of any character referred to in this book. To see more of Leah's photography, visit ldenbokphotography.com.

LESSON 10: Reconciliation with Canada's Indigenous people is an important journey. What is your first step?

The road we travel is equal in importance to the destination we seek. There are no shortcuts. When it comes to truth and reconciliation, we are all forced to go the distance."
–Justice Murray Sinclair, Chair of the Truth and Reconciliation Commission of Canada, to the Canadian Senate Standing Committee on Indigenous Peoples

I worked at a tertiary care hospital emergency room in Winnipeg for five years. That was between 1986 and 1990, long before any talk about the Truth and Reconciliation Commission struck by the Canadian government to address the historical terror faced by Canada's Indigenous people. Although educated in Canada, I had never heard of the systemic efforts in our country to eliminate Indigenous people's culture. I had no idea how this nightmare had contributed to the poverty, addiction and homelessness of so many of my Indigenous patients. It made my heart ache to see so many Indigenous people in the hospital, suffering from substance abuse and in trouble with the legal system.

I can remember a Christmas Eve shift in the Emergency Department when I was an intern. My first patient was an intoxicated Indigenous man who had a large scalp laceration. My job was to suture his wound. As I approached him, it was evident he had passed out. I tried to let him know that I was going to be sewing up his wound when he lifted up his head and spat in my face. This was repeated several times until a police officer stepped in to hold his head down so I could repair the oozing laceration.

My next patient was a young Indigenous woman who had been brought in to the Emergency Room after swallowing a large number of anti-depressants in a suicide attempt. Back in 1985, we performed an intervention known as "gastric lavage" – pumping the stomach - for patients who had overdosed. This involved placing a large bore plastic tube down the patient's throat, filling the stomach with water and then draining it out, in an attempt to wash out all of the pills prior to their absorption. The next step was the administration of activated charcoal down the tube. This was a thick slurry of black liquid that absorbed any residual medication the patient had consumed. It was an awful ritual, particularly if the patient was combative and resented your interference with their efforts to end their life. Holding the tube down the patient's throat while they cursed you and writhed in anguish was a terrible ordeal. I had three such patients that Christmas Eve. I felt like I was working in a war zone against an unknown enemy. I went home to my white privilege at 8 a.m. on Christmas morning, stunned by what I had experienced. It was impossible to process the suffering I had seen, particularly as I opened gifts with my family. Celebrating in the wake of that suffering felt so discordant, like I was betraying those patients. Some things don't compartmentalize easily.

I had no clue what was driving these Indigenous people to despair. The facts about residential schools, the separation of families, the suppression of Indigenous values, and what some have called a genocide were not discussed at all in our education system or society at large. No one at the hospital seemed to know about this historical trauma. Decades later, as the horrible truths emerged, I began to understand the torment experienced by these people and at least some of the factors that contributed to their troubled lives. I had a patient at the Mission who communicated these inconvenient truths to me in a way I will not forget.

Her name was Rita. She was in her mid-thirties and looked healthy. Tall and broad shouldered, she was a powerful presence in the examining room. Her entrance complaint was simple but would lead to a remarkably complicated encounter. "Doc, I just need something to help me with my nerves." She was new to the city, having recently come to Winnipeg from a northern Indigenous community. She was having trouble coping with city life and was sleeping at Siloam with hundreds of other people in the massive night facility. Rita wondered if I could simply give her "Valium or some Xanax" to help her relax. In the wake of my embarrassment with Jerome, I informed her that I didn't prescribe those medications at the Mission. I explained to her that drugs like valium were addictive and that I had recently had a patient who diverted the drugs to people on the street. I also told her that these types of medications don't do anything for the underlying problems that drive one's anxiety. I asked what was bothering her the most. Perhaps I could help just by offering her a listening ear. That question was like the breaking of an emotional dam, giving way to a tsunami of tears.

Rita began to weep with a deep, guttural agony that made her body convulse. She wept and she wept. Her most recent crisis was with Child and Family Services which had taken custody of her babies. This was causing her great despair. She wanted her children back. Rita's partner had died the previous year, killed by drugs. He was another victim of the fentanyl epidemic. She was overcome by grief in dealing with his passing and had turned to drugs and alcohol to cope. Her erratic behavior from the substance abuse had cost her the children; Child and Family Services had deemed her an unfit mother. She was on anti-depressants and had thoughts of killing herself. She continued to weep. I had nothing of consequence for her. How does one stem the tide of a tsunami of pain and suffering with a stethoscope?

The Truth and Reconciliation Commission of Canada began its investigations in June 2013 and released its final report in December of 2015. (18) That report was on my mind. The Truth and Reconciliation Commission documented the health disparities facing Indigenous Peoples, due in part to the ongoing intergenerational trauma caused by residential schools. Compared to non-Indigenous populations, First Nations, Métis and Inuit peoples have higher rates of diabetes, tuberculosis, cardio-respiratory and gastro-intestinal disorders, as well as higher rates of infant mortality. These negative health factors all contribute to homelessness which, in turn, leads to poor health. A downward spiral.

The Truth and Reconciliation Commission found that many survivors of residential schools developed addictions in their efforts to cope with trauma. Addiction and mental health challenges are both causes and effects of homelessness. These two factors contribute significantly to the over-representation of Indigenous Peoples living on the streets.

In clear and succinct terms, Justice Sinclair explained how our country had tried to extinguish the Indigenous culture. The fall-out was everywhere in the Indigenous community and Canadian society at large. The nearly 4,000-page document with its 94 recommendations is the culmination of a thorough investigation into Canada's residential school system that was in place between 1883 and 1969, with the final school closing only in 1996. During that time, approximately 150,000 First Nations, Métis and Inuit children were separated from their families and forced into residential schools, all across Canada. The Commission heard from 7,000 witnesses, most of whom were residential school survivors and testified to the trauma they experienced. This included physical, emotional and sexual abuse, malnutrition, disease and untimely death for many. There are reports that 3,200 children died in residential schools. The actual number may be as high as 6,000 given the poor record keeping and unmarked burial sites. (18) The findings of the Truth and Reconciliation Commission conclude that the residential school system amounted to cultural genocide:

> *Cultural genocide is the destruction of those structures and practices that allow the group to continue as a group. States that engage in cultural genocide set out to destroy the political and social institutions of the targeted group. Land is seized and populations are forcibly transferred and their movement is restricted. Languages are banned. Spiritual leaders are persecuted, spiritual practices are forbidden and objects of spiritual value are confiscated and destroyed. And, most significantly to the issue at hand, families are disrupted to prevent the transmission of cultural values and identity from one generation to*

the next. In its dealing with Aboriginal people, Canada did all these things (Truth and Reconciliation Commission, 2015:1). (18)

The cultural genocide of Canada's Indigenous Peoples and the legacy of residential schools have ongoing consequences for Indigenous Peoples today, who continue to experience systemic, institutionalized discrimination. Among its recommendations, the Truth and Reconciliation Commission proposes a public inquiry into the plight of missing and murdered Indigenous women and girls, the establishment of a National Council of Reconciliation, the enactment of an Aboriginal Languages Act, and revision of Canada's citizenship test and oath to reflect the inclusivity of Indigenous Peoples. While the final Truth and Reconciliation Commission report does not mention homelessness specifically, the legacy of residential schools has created a culture in which Indigenous Peoples are disproportionately affected by ineffective child protection policies, are over-represented in the criminal justice system, and face poorer health outcomes. Each of these factors in turn increases the likelihood that Indigenous Peoples will experience homelessness. (9) Given these realities, our country needs to develop an Indigenous homeless strategy which takes into account the findings of the Truth and Reconciliation Commission.

As I sat with Rita, I had the strangest experience. I saw a different image of the source of her tsunami of tears. It was as if her weeping was directly linked to the pain and institutional violence her people had endured. As I sat with her and watched her weep, her grief seemed to be less a response to Child and Family Services and substance abuse than to Canada's attempt to eliminate the culture of her people. While I acknowledge that our culture and environment do not exert absolute control over our destiny and that people have choices in their lives, it was clear to me that Rita had far more difficult choices that I had. I will never forget that image of a broken, sobbing Indigenous woman, suffering through so much, and how she personified clear evidence of the damage done by our government and religious institutions so many years ago.

What could I do for Rita today? I tried to comfort her. I remember praying for some inspiration about how I might help her. My human inclination to give her a hug or hold her hand was overruled by my medical training on "boundary violations." So, I simply sat with her, and repeated over and over that I could see she was suffering and that she had endured incredible traumas. It took her a long time to regain her composure. I reaffirmed that she had been through the mill. I said that any one of the tragedies she had suffered would be enough to devastate most people. We talked about getting her some counseling and regular medical care. We talked about some non-addictive sleep aids to help her navigate the Mission setting and the sleep disturbance it often exacerbates. I made sure that she had her prescription anti-depressants and reviewed with her the support options if she felt suicidal. Mostly, I just sat with her and handed her Kleenex.

Nothing in the big picture had changed for Rita. I hoped the cathartic cry had helped her feel better. She thanked me for not "just giving her pills." As she pulled herself together and got up out of her chair, she reached across the divide and gave me a hug. She said she felt a little better. I thought this would be a good place to start my reconciliation, the beginning of a process that would require "lifetimes and generations." I had been given a glimpse of the tragedy caused by residential schools in the Indigenous population. I was now aware of one source of the suffering I had observed all these years. I learned that all of our country has to start walking together toward healing. It was my first step.

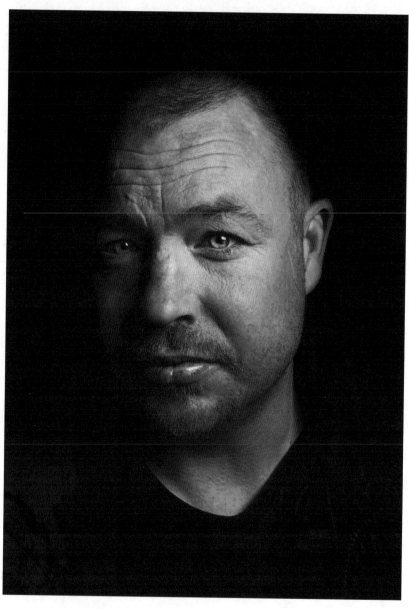

This photograph is taken with permission from Leah Denbok's work, *Nowhere to Call Home. Photographs and Stories of the Homeless. Volume One* or her website. It is not an image of any character referred to in this book. To see more of Leah's photography, visit ldenbokphotography.com.

LESSON 11:   Do not judge others by appearances, a rich heart may be under a poor coat.

—Scottish Proverb

If I stop judging others, I free myself from being judged and I can dance.
—Patti Digh

Siloam Mission has a comprehensive strategy to help people transition from life on the streets to a life of independence and dignity. The Mission has a saying that "hope begins with a meal." It is by first filling basic needs that they can help their guests begin to look to the future. Through community donations of nutritious ingredients, Siloam Mission offers 3 meals a day, 365 days a year, to as many as 400 men and women. They offer hygiene items and garments, especially warm clothes to help people through Winnipeg's notorious winters. Since May of 2007, Siloam Mission's emergency overnight shelter has offered a warm, clean, and safe environment as a place of refuge and rest for those who have no bed of their own. There, guests are welcomed and provided with toiletries, washrooms, showers and fresh towels, clean linens, and a bed for the night. The shelter holds 110 beds, as well as a 5-bed family room for short-term emergency use. The Mission strives to provide shelter in an environment that promotes dignity, self-respect and growth. Siloam offers vocational rehabilitation programs through its resource center, providing a classroom, computer lab, art program, recovery meetings, game activities, movie club, workshops, training sessions and computer workshops.

Much of Siloam's strength comes from its volunteers. In the health care center, volunteers serve in medical care, dentistry, optometry, chiropractic, physiotherapy, nursing, foot health, dental hygiene and massage therapy, as well as other disciplines. The health care center has affiliations with many professional organizations that provide service to clients in need. The volunteers show their kindness, dedication and care.

I am a fairly big guy, standing close to 6'3" and weighing over 200 pounds. This affords me a sense of confidence when dealing with some of the clients of the Mission who are agitated or come with behavioral habits learned in gangs or prison. In 34 years of practice, I have never had an altercation with a patient. By contrast, Faith is a petite, young physiotherapist who has to rely on kindness and capability. She seemed unflappable to me: calm, cool and collected, and weighing 110 pounds at most. We shared the Friday morning shift at the Mission. The physiotherapy treatment room is isolated at the back of the clinic, far away from the front desk and main office space. This arrangement never seemed to bother Faith as she escorted her patients back there for treatment. She never complained about smell, poor hygiene or other unique attributes of the homeless population. Her courage, confidence, professionalism and heart for service was inspiring.

The clinic chiropractor is also a faithful servant. Every Thursday night, Chris comes in just after supper. He knows many of the clients by name, and they appreciate the help he gives them. He has a joyful spirit and brings positive energy to the clinic. By definition, the chiropractor touches his patients. Chris touches without gloves, even though latex gloves are recommended as part of "universal blood and body fluid precautions" in health care. I began my practice before these precautions were developed and, while I understand their importance, I have always been concerned that they lessen the value of healing by touch. There is something sacred about being given the privilege of touching another person with the aim of healing. Chris's engagement and faithfulness are impressive. He is there week in and week out, providing a helping hand to people who are in pain.

Cam, another medical doctor, serves just about every Wednesday morning. He has a background in emergency medicine in an urban setting, so knows how to deal with the complexity of patient complaints in the Mission. He has the most delightful attitude - kind, caring and non-judgmental. Cam provides the bulk of medical care at the Mission but, unlike me, he is not a humble bragger. He doesn't serve for attention or accolades. He serves to help people.

There are so many volunteers, it can be difficult to keep track of them all.

One Friday morning I saw a patient I was shocked to find had fallen into the ranks of the homeless. Michael was my age and, like me, a Caucasian guy from the suburbs. He had been a successful manager at a prominent local restaurant and we had worked together over 30 years ago, he in management and me as a waiter. I immediately recognized him when he came into the clinic for sutures on his hand. I was informed that Michael was one of the people who had been working in the food preparation area and had cut his hand on a large knife. People at Siloam who are beginning to get their lives back on track are given the opportunity to re-establish work habits and to serve there, often in food prep. Michael's head was covered with a hair net to comply with food preparation requirements and he was in an old pair of jeans and a stained sweatshirt. He didn't look like the dashing executive I remembered. I was so surprised to see him. As with Lance, the basketball player from my youth, Michael was one of those guys who seemed to glide through life. He was bright, articulate and related well to people. I didn't ask him how he had ended up at a homeless mission. I suspected the probable path was drug use, an inherent risk of the party life often associated with restaurant culture. It was not for me to know.

Michael was happy to see me and didn't seem to carry any guilt or shame about his lot in life. He fondly reminisced about our time working together at the restaurant. I was worried he would feel embarrassed being on the receiving end of care in a homeless shelter but he showed no signs of discomfort. Our visit was pleasant, and he even remembered Kate and asked after her. He inquired about my life and seemed to have changed very little. I concluded that he was probably in recovery at the time, free of the effects of his addiction. I was thankful for his turn-around.

Michael's laceration required some attention. I switched back into doctor mode and starting repairing the wound. The *"It's a small world"* jingle kept coming back to me as I contemplated seeing two people from my past, both now homeless and at the same mission, within a matter of months. Michael denied any history of medical problems or any substance abuse as I completed my medical assessment. I didn't press him on the drug use, understanding he probably just wanted to get things over with as soon as possible. His past indiscretions would not interfere with the healing of a bad cut.

We finished up bandaging his wound and I gave him a handshake and wished him well. He was grateful for my attention and thanked me for volunteering at the Mission. His grasp was firm and gave me the impression that he still had an inner strength and would be able to successfully navigate his future into recovery. I felt the regrettable sense of pride at looking after this former captain of industry, thankful that my life had not ventured into the abyss as his did.

Later that morning, I shared with Angelika my amazement at seeing another old friend in the ranks of the homeless. She asked who I was referring to and I told her about Michael. She looked confused and explained that Michael was an executive from a large multi-national corporation who was volunteering in food preparation services at Siloam for the entire week. He was leading a corporate challenge of giving back to the community. He had been interviewed on the radio that very morning! I felt so embarrassed as I reflected on my condescending attitude towards the man. Yikes. Michael was a good guy doing a good work for others and I had cast him in the role of a recovering addict. How dare I? Schadenfreude? My smug feeling of superiority reminded me of my pride problem.

Condescension is a common plight for homeless people. They are often treated with judgment and disdain as they poke through the trash or ask for help on the street. The affluent so often fail to see the thin line that separates the haves from the have nots. Michael taught me the truth of the Scottish proverb: be careful of judging by appearances; a rich heart may be under a poor coat—or for that matter, a hair net.

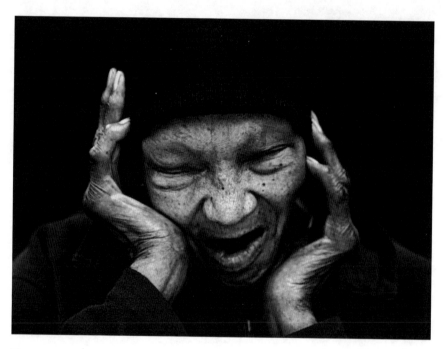

This photograph is taken with permission from Leah Denbok's work, *Nowhere to Call Home. Photographs and Stories of the Homeless. Volume One* or her website. It is not an image of any character referred to in this book. To see more of Leah's photography, visit ldenbokphotography.com.

LESSON 12: If I want to follow Jesus, I need to wash people's feet. To wash people's feet, I need to get on my knees.

To touch is to heal
To hurt is to steal
If you want to kiss the sky
Better learn how to kneel (on your knees boy!)
—U2: Mysterious Ways

One of the most potently-recurring images of my time at the Siloam clinic is providing care to people with foot problems. This is particularly ironic because, in first year medical school, my anatomy partner and I decided that the foot was too complicated to learn in the time available, so we took a chance and didn't dissect that part of the body at all. We figured there would only be one question about the foot on the exam but that we would have to spend too much valuable time to understand the complexity of this design marvel. We were right, just one question regarding the foot was set on the exam, and we saved ourselves hours and hours of memorization. Lest this make you question my competence or dismiss me as a complete fraud, I can reassure you that I have since made up for this glaring omission in my early training. I studied the foot extensively during my sports medicine fellowship and, in fact, demonstrated the dissection for the medical students at the University of British Columbia in the second year of my Master's degree there. Better late than never.

People who live on the street are on their feet most of the day. They walk to get to appointments, walk to stay warm, and walk because people don't want them loitering in one spot for too long. All this trekking around is typically done in second-hand footwear that doesn't fit properly. The additional burdens of diseases like diabetes and alcohol use disorder cause damage to peripheral nerves, making skin prone to blisters, ulcers and infections. This, combined with sweating, old socks and the lack of regular bathing, makes foot problems one of the most common entrance complaints at the Mission clinic. Siloam is well-served by a foot nurse and donated supplies from Canadian Footwear, a local shoe store that specializes in treating foot pathology through appropriate footwear. I recall my interactions with several patients where the example of Jesus washing his disciples' feet helped me provide care with a positive attitude, despite the many challenges encountered in this line of work.

Brandy was an Indigenous woman in her mid-thirties. She wanted to get clearance for "detox", a process through which a client is medically examined and found to be at low risk to go through withdrawal of drugs or alcohol. Brandy had been drinking—mostly beer but up to 20 a day—for the past several months. This level of alcohol intake would be enough to lead to potential withdrawal two or three days after she stopped drinking. Brandy had not experienced alcohol withdrawal previously, nor did she have any other risk factors for the withdrawal process.

Alcohol withdrawal is associated with many potential threats to the health of the individual. The patient may become very agitated, with profound sympathetic nervous system activation that leads to high blood pressure, a rapid heart rate and tremulousness. Even mild alcohol withdrawal can be very unpleasant. The person going through more severe withdrawal from alcohol can become delirious and experience convulsions. The Delirium Tremens—DT's—is a very serious condition characterized by intense tremulousness, agitation, dangerously high blood pressure and total disorientation, often with hallucinations. I had seen a great deal of this in my prior work at the Health Sciences Center, which had the only in-patient Chemical Withdrawal Unit in the province. It was my job to assess Brandy for her journey ahead.

Brandy looked as if she would be able to begin the withdrawal process at a local non-medical detoxification center and we completed the paper work. As we chatted, Brandy brought up some more medical concerns. Despite telling me that she had no medical problems besides alcohol, she wanted to ask me about a bad rash she had. She rolled up her pants and showed me her legs. They were covered in blood-soaked fragments of toilet paper. The paper was matted down on her skin, and in tatters. I couldn't think of a worse way to dress weeping leg wounds, but people who live on the streets are remarkably tough and make do with what they have. I often contrast their attitudes with those of the affluent people I see in my sport medicine clinic and with my own neediness as a patient when I detect some new ache or pain. I'm off to my doctor like a shot if my knee hurts after I ride my fancy bicycle a hundred miles in a week. Don't get me wrong: all pain is real, all suffering worth trying to eradicate, and the affluent among us are as entitled to medical care as anyone else. But the ailment intolerance of mainstream society is put into proper perspective by the challenges the homeless endure. To call these people resilient is an understatement.

We had to slowly soak the paper and peel it off so as not to disturb the underlying skin. Her legs and feet were covered with a weepy red friable rash. Areas of superficial infection were surrounded by excoriations from scratching and chafing. It didn't look serious enough to require hospitalization, but it looked incredibly uncomfortable. I didn't have a clue what it was. I wondered about something called guttate psoriasis, where multiple circular patches develop on the legs. I felt better when Brandy told me that the dermatologist didn't know what it was either. There was no blockage in her circulatory system, no obvious neurological anomaly I could detect, and she was not toxic, having a normal temperature and vital signs. I told her that I would bandage her up with better dressings and refer her to another dermatologist.

I have tried to conceptualize the foot care process at the Mission as a sacred rite. I think of Jesus intentionally washing his disciple's feet. (19) The symbolism of this act demonstrates that the community that Jesus called together is to manifest the love of God through serving one another, with no vestige of pride or position. Cleaning people's feet is a good place to start. Jesus said if you are to be great, you must be a servant. (20)

Being in a room with a homeless person and carefully wrapping pristine dressings on their battered feet brings me a curious sort of joy. Brandy watched closely as I used some scissors and forceps to debride some dead skin from her legs and cleansed her feet with sterile saline; I mused that Jesus would not have had this specialized solution. I then applied a topical antibiotic cream to treat some of the superficial infections, and Brandy said that the cool cream felt good against her inflamed legs. Non-adherent pads were the next step, and these light sterile products looked so good compared to the toilet paper patches. I was thankful for the people who donate these supplies to Siloam and was reminded that there is a massive behind-the-scenes team facilitating the work of the clinic. Kerlex wraps were the final step. These soft but sturdy products allow some swelling in the leg to come and go and are very comfortable. Brandy was very happy with her freshly dressed legs, although I doubt she experienced anything of the sacred as I had. I wished her well on her journey to the detox center. I knew the recidivism rate was high for people struggling with alcohol and, deep down, I expected to see her again.

Not all patients at the clinic who need their feet attended to evoke such a sense of empathy. Some are larger than life and make you laugh. Melvin was a big Indigenous man from a northern reserve, probably standing 6'6" and weighing close to 300 lbs. He had a dry sense of humor and was very playful as I asked him how I could help. One liners, double entendres, and good old-fashioned slapstick were his style of humor. He was quite matter-of-fact about having had "too much fun in the last two weeks in all the wrong places and in all the wrong shoes." He had been partying in the city over the last while and had obtained a pair of shoes from the Mission that were good looking but poorly fitting. He trotted out the old line, "It's better to look good than feel good." His feet were a mess. Massive blisters with secondary infection enveloped his ankles and feet. He informed me that he was diabetic and hadn't been paying attention to his blood sugars. We checked, and his glucose level was 16—high but not dangerous in the short term but providing a great medium for bacteria to grow. He acknowledged that he had to take better care of himself.

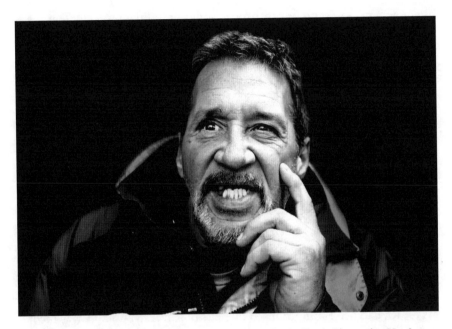

This photograph is taken with permission from Leah Denbok's work, *Nowhere to Call Home. Photographs and Stories of the Homeless. Volume One* or her website. It is not an image of any character referred to in this book. To see more of Leah's photography, visit ldenbokphotography.com.

Melvin's repertoire of one-liners made it easy to enjoy the sacred ritual of cleaning his feet. He found it was hilarious that I had to put up with his "Longfellows that smelled like the Dickens", a quote my father had used decades ago. His blisters needed to be debrided and dressed with an antibiotic cream. The process was just as it had been with Brandy and, like her, Melvin watched carefully as I cleaned and dressed his feet. He regaled me with humorous anecdotes about his recent experiences and his life in general. He sang Garth Brooks songs and did a respectable impersonation of the country music icon. He was disappointed when I told him he wouldn't be dancing for a while. I was able to get him some fresh socks, again donated by supporters of the Mission, and a pair of better fitting shoes.

Melvin gave me a remarkably solid fist bump as we finished the visit, and quipped that my sense of smell was probably ruined. I told him that foot odor was an occupational hazard and that I would be billing time and a half for him, a sort of danger pay. I recycled my line that I didn't do pedicures or manicures. He gave a big belly laugh and walked out, padding gingerly on his twinkle toes.

Not all the foot washing experiences are so gratifying. John was an Indigenous man in his mid-thirties, with a youthful appearance despite a myriad of scars criss-crossing his face. I could see he was tired and in pain. His garbled speech made him difficult to understand. It turned out that his health had been compromised by years of solvent abuse. He was incontinent of urine and one of the worst-smelling patients I have ever treated.

Solvent abusers often have a remarkably jovial affect but not this man. He was almost expressionless as he told me about the burns on his feet. A cigarette had dropped from his hands after he had fallen asleep in his Main Street hotel. Having spilled some solvent on his legs, they had been engulfed in flames. John had sustained extensive partial and full thickness burns to both of his feet. This accounted for his shuffling and arduous gait. He had not been getting regular dressing changes and dirty, unraveling gauze provided little in terms of protection for his vulnerable skin. John needed the foot washing ritual, but the odor of urine, infection and solvents was overwhelming. I knew I would need supernatural help to work through this and reflected on the image of Jesus washing his disciple's feet for motivation.

The dressing ritual began again: saline rinse, gentle cleaning of the feet, careful debridement of dead skin, application of antibiotic burn cream and gauze wrapping. John didn't want to talk and fell asleep on the examination table as I attended to his feet. I wondered what was going through his mind. Was pain his dominant emotion? What was he trying to forget? Did he view me as a helper, or as part of the colonizing enemy that had tried to destroy his people? I tapped him on the shoulder when I was finished with his dressings. He said "Thanks Doc" and left the treatment room as quietly as he had entered it. He had no home to go back to. He couldn't recline and elevate his feet, allowing his pain and swelling to abate. He would be forced out into the cold, to walk the mean streets as he tried to keep his dressings clean and dry. I hoped the dressings would last through the next few days, time that would almost certainly be clouded by sniffing toxins, profound sadness and pain.

How people like John survive amazes me. I and my affluent peers rely on vitamins, supplements, protein shakes, Greek yogurt, and organic gluten free diets, with boot camp, yoga or a spin class for health. We make sure we have every angle covered to guarantee we are fit and strong. This man reminded me just how much punishment a human can take and still put one foot in front of the other - even if the feet are burned, infected and painful. I have found that the longer I practice at Siloam, the more I actually look forward to washing people's feet. Some would say I need to get out more.

Jane was in her late twenties and of Metis heritage. She had the most mesmerizing green eyes. She trudged into the examination room carrying a big hockey bag full of all her belongings. She had two winter coats to deal with the frigid winter temperatures. She was worried about her feet as her second-hand boots didn't fit well and she had painful blisters. As we talked about her feet, she told me of her many troubles.

Jane was on probation, having been charged with assault. She was trying to remain abstinent from Xanax (a benzodiazepine) and cannabis and had found that she was easily agitated. She had been in several fights at another shelter and had been evicted. She grew up in northern Manitoba but had been raised in the Child and Family Services system. She was matter-of-fact about her life challenges and some of her victories as well. She acknowledged having a pre-disposition to addiction and had good insight into the negative role cannabis had played in her life. Jane said that despite being *high* for the better part of two years, she said she felt remarkably *low*. She was living proof that cannabis is addictive and often destructive. Jane had begun working with a counsellor and was being honest with herself for the first time in her life. She had a difficult time explaining what that meant, but we both saw it as something good.

Jane's feet were in rough shape. Wet and badly worn socks covered infected blisters which were caked with dirt. She needed the treatment. As she lay back on the examining table she told me how much better she felt being drug-free. She described a clarity of thought and purpose she had never experienced. She giggled as I cleaned the dirt out from between her toes with a cotton swab. She would require some minor debridement of the infected areas and I had to leave the room to get the equipment. When I returned, she was fast asleep, taking advantage of the brief period of calm that the Mission can provide amidst the chaos of the street. It was difficult for me to relate to just how tired she must have been. I washed her feet in that oasis of peace.

Sparrow was a twenty-something Caucasian female. Before I saw her, Angelika came back to the examining room and warned me that she might be a tough patient. She sat in the waiting room with wearing a flamboyant hat, a wild tie-dye muscle shirt and tattooed profanities on her arms. She was talking very loudly and had the attention of the entire waiting room, full of tired people waiting to see the doctor. Evidently no detail of her life was considered private, as she shared remarkably personal information with her captive audience. I was prepared for some foot washing, as the nurse's note from the day before detailed badly blistered feet that required dressing and perhaps antibiotics.

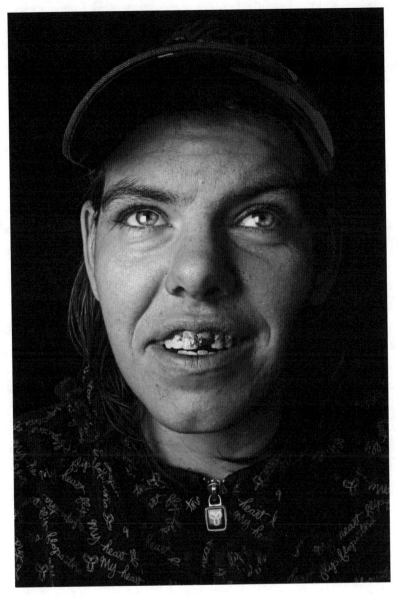

This photograph is taken with permission from Leah Denbok's work, *Nowhere to Call Home. Photographs and Stories of the Homeless. Volume One* or her website. It is not an image of any character referred to in this book. To see more of Leah's photography, visit ldenbokphotography.com.

Sparrow sounded awful when she came into the examining room. She had a very noisy cough and a hoarse voice. Before I could introduce myself, she said that she needed a lot of help. She was sore from head to toe. She was worried about her lungs and her feet in particular. As I started to ask some questions, she said she had borderline personality disorder and depression after a long history of sexual abuse. I didn't know what to say, as very few patients are that blunt in their first few sentences. Something in me said "go to her feet." I asked her if I could see her feet, and she took off her socks and laid down on the examining table. Her blisters were not very serious and, thankfully, were not infected. However, her feet had dirt ground into them so deeply it resembled another tattoo. I asked her if I could wash her feet. She seemed pleased at this prospect and I started doing my best to clean off the grime. I hadn't planned this but it gave us a chance to develop some trust, which was particularly important given her past history of abuse. I got her feet as clean as I could and then put a moisturizing cream on them. The whole procedure took about ten minutes and through that entire time she told me about her troubled life. The tapestry of family of origin abuse, depression, drug use and eventual homelessness were the central features of her journey. As I listened her story, it was remarkable how strong she seemed despite all the trauma she had been through.

Once we finished with Sparrow's feet it was time to deal with her bad cough. Her vital signs were fine, and that was re-assuring. Her lungs sounded terrible, with scattered loud wheezes throughout, as well as an area with diminished breath sounds, which signaled potential pneumonia. She didn't think she had HIV or any of the serious illnesses that could compromise her immune system, so I thought we could treat her as an outpatient. I told her I wanted to get an x-ray of her chest and was surprised at how thankful she was for that basic investigation. I prescribed her an antibiotic and a combination puffer to help with her wheezing. I was worried about her as she headed out into the reality of the street. Would she get her medications? Would she get her x-ray? Would she be safe?

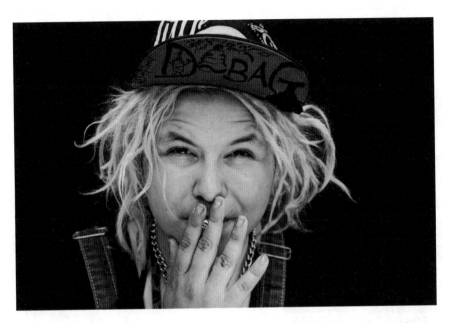

This photograph is taken with permission from Leah Denbok's work, *Nowhere to Call Home. Photographs and Stories of the Homeless. Volume One* or her website. It is not an image of any character referred to in this book. To see more of Leah's photography, visit ldenbokphotography.com.

At my next shift one week later, Sparrow was on the list of patients. She looked completely different. The flamboyant hat replaced by a dark toque, and her top a simple hoody. I was happy to see her, and thankful that her breathing appeared easier. Her respiratory condition had improved but was still far from normal. She had a good laugh at my expense as, apparently, I was in big trouble. I hadn't charted that I washed her feet and put cream on them during her last visit. As a consequence of my oversight, when Sparrow had been in the clinic the day before, asking the nurse for some more of the cream and a foot rub, they thought she was making the whole thing up. I was also in trouble because she told Angelika that I had given her alcohol swabs to wash her feet. I had found that the alcohol was more effective than soap. It was news to me that this was a clinic no-no, as some desperate people will actually squeeze the non-beverage alcohol out of the swabs and drink it. I think the fact that I was in trouble cemented our relationship. Sparrow had not been for her x-ray, so I tried to convince her that it was not elective and that I was concerned about significant lung pathology. Angelika encouraged her as well. She agreed to get it done and commented that this might have been the first time anyone was really concerned for her.

One foot-washing experience was particularly heart-wrenching but exemplified the good work the Mission can do. Bruce was a young man from Vietnam. He had a very slight build and looked to be about 12 years old. In fact, he was 21, the age of my son. His family had immigrated to Canada years ago. He had been kicked out of his parent's home for reasons he did not want to discuss. He found himself living on the street. He had all his belongings in three duffle bags and presented to the Mission clinic in very agitated state. He was having chest pain and felt like he was going to throw up.

Providentially, Bruce was assessed by Lea, a naturopath who was working with me that morning. Lea had worked for Naturopaths Without Borders and participated in several service trips to Haiti and Mexico. She was hoping to provide services at Siloam, and I had been showing her some of the ropes. A female presence was helpful in calming Bruce down. He had been sleeping under a bridge for a week or so but had needed a few nights inside. He had attended another mission organization earlier in the week and had been sleeping in a dorm room with eight men. The previous night, Bruce had awoken to find one of the men sexually assaulting him. He was then threatened with death if he told anyone of the incident. He was having a full-blown panic attack, literally shaking from head to toe.

Bruce thought he was having a heart attack and was freaking out. He couldn't stop moving. To make matters worse, he was covered with bed bug bites. His appearance and emotional state broke our hearts. Lea was able to reassure him that his heart and lungs were fine, with normal vital signs and a normal clinical exam. Bruce was worried about where he could go, feeling that all avenues for him had been closed. As he contemplated more time on the street, he told us that his feet were badly blistered by his work boots. Despite sleeping under a bridge, he was managing to hold down a construction job and worried that his foot trouble was going to prevent him from working. Lea asked me to assess his feet to see if he needed antibiotics, as that was outside the scope of her naturopath practice. That's when I thought that Bruce needed the foot washing ritual.

I asked him if I could wash his feet, and he seemed shocked. He agreed they needed it, given he had not had access to bathing facilities for several days. I had him lie down and I think he started to calm down for the first time. I got some gauze and sterile water and cleaned the grime off the blisters. With all that this young man had been through, he really needed some simple kindness. As I was working on his feet, Bruce uttered a heartfelt "Thank you." He didn't need antibiotics, but we were able to give him some nice new socks which were greatly appreciated.

When we finished our time with Bruce, I asked Angelika to see if he could be given a room for respite for the rest of the day. The Mission has a family room for this purpose and, as luck would have it, it had just opened up. He would be safe and sound for the next 24 hours and have a chance to begin his recovery from the traumatic events he had endured. Siloam was there, standing in the gap, providing hope. It was moving to be a part of it. Still, Bruce's experience of family alienation, homelessness and abuse was so very sad.

People like Brandy, Melvin, John, Jane, Sparrow and Bruce can be viewed from several perspectives. We can judge them as people making bad choices, who are simply suffering the consequences of their actions. We can pretend that they had a stable upbringing and have a supportive family somewhere. We can ignore that our government tried to eradicate their culture. While there is only one reality, theirs is different from most of ours. From a judgmental vantage point, we decide that people get what they deserve: you live on the street because of your poor choices. Sadly, judgment often leads to condemnation.

We can also view suffering people through the lens of mercy. People can be spared from suffering the full consequences of their behavior. Siloam Mission is clearly a place of mercy, where people are protected from the cold and lonely world of the streets. Most of the time, we never speak to the patients about how they became homeless. The Mission is not there to cast blame. The only time mercy may not be warranted is in the area of co-dependence. This involves a well-meaning giver of mercy protecting their loved one from the consequences of their bad choices, to the point where the damaging behavior is enabled, continues and may worsen. The co-dependent covers up for the alcoholic so that the person's behavior doesn't embarrass them or their family. The alcoholism continues. Co-dependence can perpetuate the behavior and ultimately cause more trouble.

We can also serve people through the filter of grace. Grace is shown in circumstances where people are given a gift they may not deserve. Bad choices are acknowledged, and their role in leading to one's suffering have to be explored. But grace involves a spirit of benevolence and kindness, giving people a chance to move in a new direction. One of the things I love most about the Mission is that you see grace unfurled on a regular basis. The homeless reduction movement believes that people are helped the most by giving them a place to live. Don't wait until a needy person gets sober and healthy before putting a roof over his or her head. When the person on the street finds a home, the evidence indicates he or she is more likely to get well and sober.

Judgment: You get what you deserve.
Mercy: You don't get what you deserve.
Grace: You get something you don't deserve. (21)

It seems to me that mercy and grace beat judgment every time.

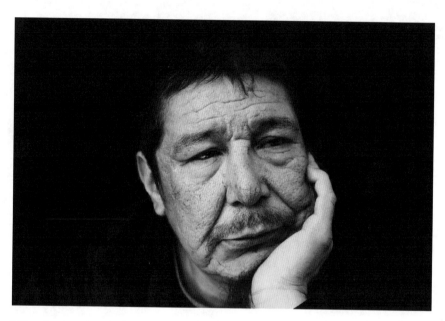

This photograph is taken with permission from Leah Denbok's work, *Nowhere to Call Home. Photographs and Stories of the Homeless. Volume One* or her website. It is not an image of any character referred to in this book. To see more of Leah's photography, visit ldenbokphotography.com.

LESSON 13: It's good to cry. You need to get tears out because they cause rust if left inside.

When people kill themselves, they think they're ending the pain,
but all they're doing is passing it on to those they leave behind.
—*Jeannette Walls*

A sense of satisfaction at the Mission can come from working on hands as well as feet. Martin was an Indigenous man in his late twenties. The infection on his hand was just the tip of the iceberg of his troubled life. Martin was thin and wiry and was unemotional as he showed me his badly-infected hand. He wasn't sure what had happened. He had been on a week-long drinking binge and noticed an abscess forming in his palm. He had a scab over his knuckles and suspected that he may have punched somebody in the mouth, cutting the skin on his combatant's teeth. Such wounds are treated as human bites, which have a high risk of infection by anaerobic bacteria that can be difficult to eradicate.

The abscess was angry and would have to be incised and drained. I asked Martin if he had any other medical problems that might make him more susceptible to infection, and he thought not. He did have many troubles, some medical, some emotional. He was on methadone, an opioid given to people who have been addicted to that class of medications. He was taking valium, an old-school benzodiazepine that is a potent sedative/anxiolytic. He was also taking Wellbutrin, a newer generation anti-depressant.

I asked him if he wanted to talk about his troubles as we prepared to drain the abscess in his hand. The flood gates opened.

Martin had become hooked on opioids at a young age. The usual story. Partying, first with pills from family members' medicine cabinets, then buying more powerful drugs on the street, then the intravenous use of anything that would get him high. The process took only a few years, but left Martin homeless and alienated from friends and family. His depression and anxiety were related to the legacy of drugs in his life but, more recently, his baby sister had committed suicide on the reserve. He then told me the incredible saga of death in his family of origin. His father died violently, and his mother also died from suicide. His brother died while in the penitentiary. And then his baby sister. Martin started to weep as he reflected on all these tragedies. I handed him a tissue and told him that it was good to cry, because the tears caused rust if left on the inside. He was able to manage a thin smile through his tears.

I know too well the trauma inflicted upon a family by suicide. My brother, Bill, died at his own hand. At 21, my brother became depressed. I was just 11 at the time. My older sisters believe he had endured a bad experience with LSD and that it estranged him from his group of friends. He had hoped to be a pilot but the job prospects in the early 1970's were bleak and there was some question of whether the acid trip had shut the door to flying. Bill's heart was not in his university studies of psychology and philosophy. I can remember him ruminating over the philosophical premise, "God is dead." The final straw was when a young woman used him to make her boyfriend jealous.

Bill's first suicide attempt involved overdosing on tranquilizers. I found him "asleep" at the kitchen table when I came home from school. The house was quiet and there was a candle burning in front of him. He had rested his head on his arms atop the table. I remember there was a cake I wasn't supposed to eat before dinner, and I thought Bill was feigning sleep to catch me at my predictable fridge-raiding. I was astonished when he didn't even flinch as I cut myself a generous slice of cake. Much private discussion occurred between my parents that night, and I had no clue why my brother had to go to the hospital. He didn't look sick, he was just pretending to be asleep to catch me eating cake. Bill and I shared a bedroom, and his absence left me feeling vulnerable.

On the second attempt, my brother meant business. Near the end of my Grade 6 year, just my mom and I were home after school one day when she asked me to go to the basement to get some flour. It was kept in the furnace room. When I opened the door to the room, I found Bill hanging. I remember pleading with God to save him, as we waited in vain for the ambulance. I am still haunted by the image of my mom struggling with his lifeless body, trying to take him down from his improvised gallows. I was told to report to my school friends and teachers that Bill had died from a brain aneurysm.

Bill's death exploded my parents' already-toxic relationship. By the time I was in my teens, my parents were fully at war, each struggling with their own demons and the trauma of losing a child to suicide, blaming each other, blaming themselves. They were permanently scarred by the worst trauma a parent can experience.

I couldn't fathom the suffering that Martin must be enduring with so many deaths to grieve. He had found out quickly that opioids were not the solution to his problem but he was still running fast. I asked him to lie down so I could deal with the abscess in his hand. The chance to recline seemed to be a welcome respite from the stress and mayhem of his life on the street. Martin's hand was filthy and would need a thorough cleansing before we opened up the abscess to drain the pus, a necessary step in the treatment of these wounds. I had felt the sacred ritual of washing many people's feet in the clinic before but washing Martin's hand was different.

The young man had been to hell and back and was still suffering. Once again, the difference between Martin and me was so evident. This striking contrast is an aspect of my life and my sport medicine practice that makes me feel a sense of shame. Like so many others, I have invested far too much time and energy in obsessive physical training, and my body pays the price. It hurts when I train for a marathon. I have hip pain when I do my adventure races. I wonder to myself, do these things fall under the category of "small minded and lop-sided pursuits" referred to in Eugene Peterson's scripture rendering, *The Message*? Peterson describes such pursuits as reflective of trying to get our own way all the time, a focus on self at the expense of the other. (1) I am guilty of this. I am an obsessive exerciser, constantly worried about being fit and winning the competition with illusory rivals. If I don't do 1000 push-ups a week, I'm falling behind. I wonder what our world would look like if a small portion of the time, energy and money we all invest in our *fitness* was diverted to the less fortunate. I have seen so many unhappy exercise enthusiasts in my practice. I sometimes ask patients who seem trapped in an obsession with exercise and have trained themselves into ill-health, "What are you running from?" I have asked that question of myself many times.

I became obsessed with endurance training during a period when Kate and I had split-up before we were married. We had parted ways after dating for five years, mostly because I couldn't commit to marriage. To me, with my family of origin experiences, marriage looked like a brutal institution. Marriage was toxic. Running was a great way to process my emotions, stay fit and deal with free time. To be honest, I think I was running from loneliness and insecurity. I was running from embarrassment at being single. Soon, given my predilection, I ran for pride. I felt better, and I could compete with others. How fast was that mile? I ran from my fears for several years until Kate and I decided to each get some counselling on our relationship, which had stalled into a limbo where we couldn't commit to each other but couldn't let go either. I ran my way right into the office of an Anglican Priest who was able to help me with my fear of marital commitment.

According to my agenda, my counsellor was supposed to aid me in my relationship with Kate and help me cope with all of her faults (ok, the one fault). To my frustration, he just kept asking me about my family. What was my relationship like with my dad, my mom? What was their relationship like? When he asked me about my siblings, I was surprised to discover the ocean of tears I had dammed up about the loss of my brother. I probably wept for 15 minutes, deep racking sobs that caught me totally off-guard. I was embarrassed, but my counsellor was calm and patient and offered me the wisdom I have since passed on to others. As I struggled vainly to pull myself together, he handed me a tissue and said, "It's good to cry; you need to get tears out because they cause rust if you leave them on the inside." Over a series of sessions, my Anglican friend taught me that the dysfunction in my family's past did not predestine me to failure in my future family life. The cycle could be broken. There was hope for my relationship with Kate. None of the big problems were hers. They were all mine, all rooted in my family of origin troubles. He taught me that you can break the chain of family of origin dysfunction. It changed my life.

Martin's hand was very inflamed, so I tried to be as gentle as possible as I drained the abscess in his palm. We carefully anesthetized the region and incised the abscess with a gratifying evacuation of blood and pus. Again, the dressing ritual was followed, and again, I felt its sacred nature. Treating Martin was made different by our shared experience of suicide. Martin got up from the treatment table, looked me in the eye, gave me a simple nod and left the room. I had a glimpse of the pain he must have been enduring. I saw it in his eyes. I knew that Martin would have a much harder time breaking the cycle of violence in his life. He was not just fighting his family of origin demons, but years of systemic racial discrimination and marginalization. My time with Martin underscored for me that those of us who have endured the suicide of a loved one share an unspoken bond. We mourn not only their loss but their deaths in unrelenting pain. Surely, we can find a better way to stop this pain.

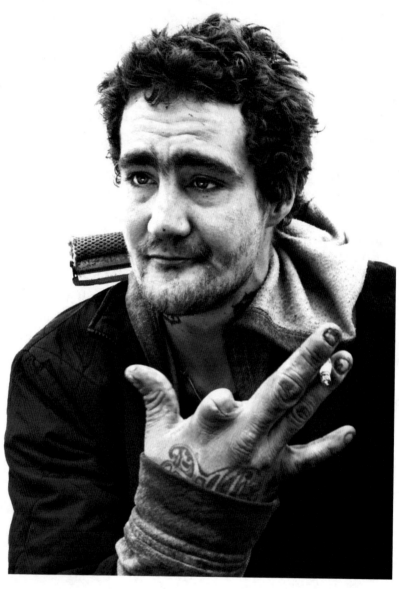

This photograph is taken with permission from Leah Denbok's work, *Nowhere to Call Home. Photographs and Stories of the Homeless. Volume One* or her website. It is not an image of any character referred to in this book. To see more of Leah's photography, visit ldenbokphotography.com.

LESSON 14:

Mental illness is not contagious. You can't catch it by lending a hand.

"Mental pain is less dramatic than physical pain, but it is more common and also more hard to bear."
—*C.S. Lewis*

People suffering from mental illness are disproportionately represented at homeless shelters. Schizophrenia, bipolar disorder, depression, anxiety, borderline personality disorder, panic, and substance use disorder afflict many of our clients. People with these conditions do not require hospitalization but can struggle to navigate lives of independence, especially if they don't take their medication. We see many people who are just starting their psychotic breaks, spiraling downward into a delusional morass, having lost their jobs and their families, but not yet at a point where they are a danger to themselves or others. They resist suggestions that they are mentally-ill and, in their paranoid delusions, people trying to help become part of the conspiracy that is out to get them.

"Insane asylums" used to house people with these illnesses. Prior to effective anti-psychotic medications, sufferers were institutionalized and chemically or physically restrained. A brief flirtation with the infamous *frontal lobotomy* and early electric shock therapy proved to be no better than the other measures. The asylums were notorious places that deserved their reputation. Ken Kesey's 1962 book, *One Flew Over the Cuckoo's Nest*, chronicled the bizarre goings-on in some of these facilities. With the advent of medications like the phenothiazines, approved by the American FDA in 1954, people with these conditions could be effectively treated and no longer required institutionalization. The process of de-institution-alization began in the 1960's, with the goal of improving the treatment of mentally-ill people while decreasing costs associated with their man-agement. In the United States, close to 500,000 people were discharged from mental health asylums in the 1960's. Unfortunately, the promise of successful medical treatment was not realized for many patients with psychotic illnesses. The streets and jails became their refuge. As of 2014, in the U.S.A., it was estimated that 2.2 million mentally-ill people did not receive any psychiatric care at all. This is thought to account for one-third of the total homeless population and close to 20% of the population in jails and prisons. The situation in Canada is marginally better, given the government-funded single payer medical system, but mentally-ill people are still disproportionately homeless and incarcerated.

As long as people with psychotic illnesses take their medications, they can lead productive lives, deal with many difficult situations and accom-plish their goals. Nate was one such fellow. He was a large Indigenous man with schizoaffective disorder, a hybrid between schizophrenia and bipolar disorder. He had very pressured speech and flight of ideas. His speech was fast and intense. Nate had jet black hair and penetrating dark eyes. Until I got to know him, I found him to be quite intimidating. He talked with his hands, which was particularly unnerving because he had lost several fingers to frostbite, another common consequence of being mentally-ill and homeless in a city like Winnipeg. The whole package was quite unset-tling. In reality, Nate was a remarkably friendly, kind and gentle person who was quick to develop loyalty.

Nate had had a remarkable string of medical difficulties. In his pres-sured manner of speech, he recounted battles with blood cancer, stomach cancer, oropharyngeal cancer and schizoaffective disorder. His cancers were probably related to smoking, an affinity many people with mental illness share. Nate's problems were always related in a matter-of-fact fashion, not as a plea for sympathy. His discourse was more like a recitation committed to memory to ensure his health care providers wouldn't overlook anything.

He ran through his medication list like an eloquent pharmacist, spelling each medication and noting the exact dosage in milligrams and frequency of administration. I am on Seroquel, S-E-R-O-Q-U-E-L, 300 mg at HS, Citalopram, C-I-T-A-L-O-P-R-A-M, 20 mg od in the a.m., etc. Nate had been my one exception for the prescription of sedative medications when his doctor was out of town. He usually brought me the doctor's phone number so I could confirm that she was away and that prescription of these medications would be appropriate. Nate was one of the success stories of a person with serious psychiatric illness who had survived without much support from family, friends or the broader medical community. I was amazed at his ability to deal with profound troubles with a positive attitude and none of the "poor me" syndrome.

I think of Nate when I start to pout over some medical problem that my hypochondriasis has invented. Like many doctors, I can be convinced I have a devastating illness by a single symptom of that disorder. Indigestion for me is always stomach cancer, never too much rich food or wine. The rash is always skin cancer, not athlete's foot. Kate will usually dismiss my concerns with a simple, "You're fine." On our honeymoon, Kate and I went to Hawaii. Back in the early 90's, tanning was still a laudable goal and we wanted to get "mahogany brown." On the first day of our vacation, I was looking at my thigh and noticed a red, irregular lesion that I was sure was a melanoma, the deadly type of skin cancer related to sun exposure. I panicked and headed for the hotel room. I started calling all of the plastic surgeons in Hawaii, wanting to have this thing removed before it spread. Between calls, I scolded Kate for her recklessness in staying in the sun. I couldn't get any appointments before our honeymoon was over. I threatened the surgeons' receptionists with lawsuits if I had to lose my leg to this dreaded lesion. They all hung up on me.

I contemplated the implications of having cancer. I got very sad very quickly. I thought of the large incision into my quadriceps that would be required to excise the tumor with a wide margin. I mused that this would end my career as a triathlete and might even threaten my independence. At low ebb and firmly in panic-mode, it finally dawned on me that I had had a biopsy of that area during my sport medicine fellowship as part of a research project. The lesion was not melanoma at all. It was a scar! I was ecstatic, and promptly joined Kate on the beach so I could work on my tan. When feeling sorry for myself for some imaginary illness, someone as tough as Nate reminds me of the character it takes to persevere through real suffering. He was tough, I was a pretender. Of the two of us, he was the real Ironman.

A tragic number of patients with mental illness have limited insight into their condition and have not been formally diagnosed. By virtue of poor impulse control, agitation and frequent paranoid delusions, these people find themselves alienated from friends, family and employers. This is when they end up on the streets and at Siloam. Their behavioral problems get them into trouble at the Mission as well, and they promptly find themselves referred to the doctor. I saw a fellow with my niece, Rachel, who exemplified this complicated scenario.

Max was in his 60's, Caucasian, well-groomed and well-dressed. He had sandy blonde hair and deep blue eyes. He reminded me of Robert Redford. He seemed out of place in the Mission clinic. He could have been a movie star or a politician. But I had been warned prior to seeing him that he was an ornery man and had been giving grief to people throughout the organization. He was angry, abusive and short-tempered. Blue language filled the air with Max in the room. The workers at Siloam can put up with a lot of guff, so for them to be voicing concern meant something substantial.

Max's entrance complaint on the electronic medical record was recorded as "chest pain", something we always treat very carefully. He entered the examination room and generally looked well. I introduced Rachel and myself and asked how we could help him. He immediately started screaming at me, exclaiming that if I had enough clinical experience, I would know what his problem was. Clearly this was going to be a challenge.

I assured Max that it was customary for the patient to tell the doctor what was bothering him and then the doctor would ask the relevant questions, examine the patient and then come up with a list of potential diagnoses. Max launched into a litany of complaints about the Mission. The food was shitty, the beds terrible, the staff incompetent. I tried to bring him back to medical issues and told him that I didn't have any control over the Mission's food and sleeping accommodations. I told Max that many people are very thankful for a bed at Siloam. He fired off a few F-sharps, rolled his eyes and turned up his pant leg. "OK", he blurted, "what's the problem here, smart guy?" I looked at his leg and said "You have some edema." Edema is the collection of fluid in the leg and can be caused by a myriad of medical disorders. Some are very benign, others as dangerous as heart or liver failure. Max was not impressed. He responded that he knew that he had edema and obviously it was a clear indication that his heart was in jeopardy. He promptly concluded that I must be a shitty diagnostician. I asked him if he had any history of heart problems, and that set him off on another blue monologue that I was incompetent like all the rest of the Mission staff. He quipped that he might complain to the College of Physicians and Surgeons about my substandard care. Max was so over-the-top that the only thing I thought we could accomplish was to show Rachel how to deal with an agitated patient.

I agreed with Max that heart trouble was one of the potential causes of leg edema, but that it was a remarkably common and non-specific sign. There are many conditions associated with leg edema. My spider sense was that Max had untreated bipolar disorder to account for his pressured speech, agitation and flight of ideas, but he refused to acknowledge any such past history. It would be unusual for a patient to have their first psychotic break in their sixties, so I persisted in my questioning. I asked him about any medications he was taking and he answered forcefully, "None." I asked him if he had ever taken any medications for his mood and again he barked, "No." "Didn't you read my file" he bellowed. I told him I had read his file, but the only entry stated that he was belligerent and demanding to see a cardiologist. When I asked about street drugs that could cause delirium and agitation, he became even more indignant. I could tell Rachel was getting twitchy with our angry patient.

I suggested to Max that we should examine him to see if he had any evidence of heart disease and that we would take his concerns seriously, including organizing tests for his heart, and other potential causes of edema. He agreed, and actually seemed thankful to have an examination.

The only problem was it was difficult to hear his heart and breath sounds over his constant yelling. Max was in pretty good shape physically with no cardio-pulmonary or neurological findings. The only finding of note was that his blood pressure was high. I told him that his pressure was up and that's when Max gave away his past medical history. He asked me what his pressure was. I informed him that it was 160/95. He said that reading was common for him and wondered if it should be treated. He asked me what medications I might consider, and I suggested a simple diuretic. Those medications are inexpensive and would have the additional benefit of helping clear his leg swelling. That's when he asked me about how a diuretic would interact with Lithium - the mood stabilizer that is exclusively used to treat bipolar disorder. Bingo. Max then acknowledged that he had taken this for years but not in the last several months. He declared that the Lithium robbed him of his true self. Since being off the Lithium, he had felt more alive, but had been fired from his job, kicked out by his spouse and ended up on the street. He said that several months prior, he had also been taking Seroquel, a newer generation anti-psychotic and sedative. He mentioned a whopping dose of 300 mg. So much for the "No medications."

It was clear that Max's agitation, anger and pressured speech were associated with an untreated manic episode. When I asked him who had prescribed the medication, he informed me that he hadn't seen his psychiatrist for several months, complaining that his "shrink" did nothing but give him pills. This conundrum plagues the manic patient population. Take drugs and feel subdued or even unwell, or go drug free for a while, feel more like yourself, and then almost certainly end up in some trouble, in jail, or in Max's case, homeless and alone. Trying not to alienate Max, I told him his blood pressure was up because of his agitation. We had to help him become less agitated. To my surprise, he agreed to start a small dose of Seroquel to control both issues and to make an appointment to see his psychiatrist. At the end of the visit, he seemed almost relieved, but he did drop an F-bomb when I asked him to limit his salt intake. Rachel and I laughed when he said he wasn't sure whether I was "Dumb or Dumber."

Rachel was clearly relieved to see Max leave. He was like a tornado. A brief visit of intensity and potential destruction. Rachel had learned further lessons from the Mission medical clinic. She learned that not all medical interactions end in hugs and miracles. She learned that docs have to serve all patients, even the ornery ones. She learned that untreated mental illness is a frequent cause of homelessness. I also think she learned that mental illness is not contagious, and that you can't catch it by lending a hand. Above all, she learned that we need to find a better way to serve these people who don't belong in institutions but have so much difficulty navigating the choppy waters of life troubled by their beautiful minds.

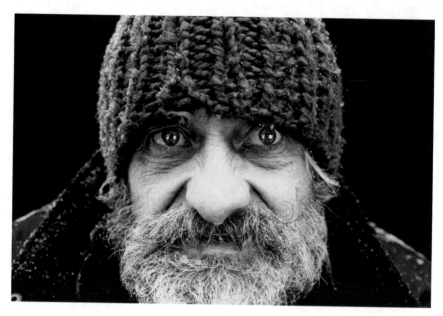

This photograph is taken with permission from Leah Denbok's work, *Nowhere to Call Home. Photographs and Stories of the Homeless. Volume One* or her website. It is not an image of any character referred to in this book. To see more of Leah's photography, visit ldenbokphotography.com.

LESSON 15: Be kind whenever possible.
It is always possible.
—the 14th Dalai Lama

The smallest act of kindness is worth more than the grandest intention.
—Oscar Wilde

Working with my niece, Rachel, is very rewarding. She picks up concepts quickly. She was able to perform blood pressure measurements and could appreciate various breath and heart sounds after her first clinic experience. She could obtain and document a complete set of vital signs in no time at all. Rachel had observed some fascinating cases, full of valuable lessons. She witnessed a miracle of provision for Sam, the blind man, and struggled through an angry interview with Max, the bipolar man who hadn't taken his medications for months. I am proud to report that Rachel has been admitted to medical school. I asked her which patient at the clinic was the most memorable for her. I was a little surprised when she said it was Paul. I couldn't think of a less dramatic patient than Paul. What had she learned from him?

Rachel and I have seen Paul at the clinic several times; in fact, he comes to most of the clinics that I have. He is an elderly Metis man who lives close to Siloam in government-supported housing. Paul is a gentle soul and he has no significant medical problems. He presents as a very meek character. You get the sense that Paul is the type of person that the world just passes by, or worse, the type that was bullied. Paul knows that I am one of the medical doctors for our storied Canadian Football League franchise, the Winnipeg Blue Bombers. Paul is an ardent fan of Winnipeg's rival, the Ottawa Redblacks, so whenever he sees me, he makes sure he has some of their team colors on. A red toque and a black scarf would be typical attire. He will always give me a little jab if the Redblacks are ahead of the Bombers in the standings and is sure to remind me of "The Drought": the fact that Winnipeg hasn't won a Grey Cup in over twenty years, the precise time-frame I have been associated with the football club. Both of us acknowledge the coincidence, Paul gleefully, me with a deep sense of melancholy. Paul was ecstatic when the Red Blacks won the Grey Cup in 2016 and was sure to remind me of this crucial fact every time we saw each other.

Paul usually presents with a medical concern involving a sore body part as his entrance complaint. After his history and physical examination, I usually tell Paul there is nothing worrisome to find and I offer him options from the usual treatment menu for his problem. He will then refuse all offerings and say that he is fine. He transitions into the football banter or some sort of playful conversation. I play along and push back a little. I remind him of a woeful season his team had in recent years. He laughs generously. He seems to enjoy his visits. I must admit I enjoy them too. If part of medicine is simply listening to your patient, expressing concern and allowing the patient to select from a list of reasonable treatment options, then I guess these can be considered medical visits.

I asked Rachel why she found Paul so noteworthy. She responded that it was the gentleness of his personality. There was no pride or arrogance or the other things that are unattractive in most of us. She also commented on the simplicity of making him "feel better." He wasn't looking for medical intervention, and we clearly didn't provide any in the conventional sense. But there was a palpable *improvement* in his demeanor after his visit. I made sure that Rachel understood that boundary issues are an important part of medical practice. I acknowledged that I relaxed the boundaries a little bit with Paul.

I believe that my relationship with Paul highlights the mysterious world of human connection at the Mission. We live in very different worlds. Paul lives alone, in poverty. I live with my family in a comfortable home in the suburbs and see hundreds of patients a month. Yet I enjoy this connection with Paul more than many other things. I respect so many of the homeless people I see for their strength in adversity, their perseverance. What I find amazing is the almost universal lack of complaining. As I have observed before, one tends to hear more complaints at the country club than the homeless shelter. With someone like Paul, kindness is easy to give and has predictably good consequences. Kindness can be so hard to come by in our world, especially if you are homeless. I wonder why we have such a hard time expressing it.

The last time I saw Paul, we engaged in the usual football banter; even in the minus 40 degree weather, he had his distinctive team colors on, a red and black toque with red and black arm bands. I asked him why he had such allegiance to the Redblacks rather than the Bombers, the Winnipeg home team. Paul said that his birth mother was from Ottawa and that is why he loves the team so dearly. He had been taken from her very early in his life. It wasn't sport fanaticism that drove his affections, it was a deep, abiding connection to his mother. It all became heartbreakingly clear. The revelation deepened my respect for this kind and gentle man. I would wear those colors too.

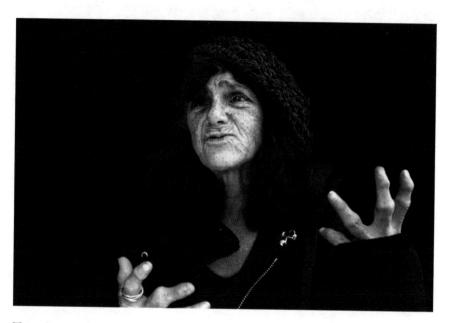

This photograph is taken with permission from Leah Denbok's work, *Nowhere to Call Home. Photographs and Stories of the Homeless. Volume One* or her website. It is not an image of any character referred to in this book. To see more of Leah's photography, visit ldenbokphotography.com.

LESSON 16: Investments in yourself are important, but investments in others can be transcendent.

There are good works waiting for you...don't be late.

For it is by grace you have been saved, through faith—and this is not from yourselves, it is the gift of God—not by works, so that no one can boast. For we are God's handiwork, created in Christ Jesus to do good works, which God prepared in advance for us to do.
—Ephesians 2: 8-10 NIV

Several years ago, I experienced a very strange series of events relating to a bicycle. I was saving money to buy a triathlon racing bike. I had full permission from Kate for this expenditure. The bike I had chosen was custom-made to conform to my unusual proportions – long legs and very short torso. It was going to cost $3000. I ordered the bike in the fall to be ready for the spring. I put down a $1000 deposit and started to stash away any cash I could to pay for it. I ended up with a wad of bright-orange Canadian fifty-dollar bills stuffed in my shaving kit that greeted me each morning as I shaved and showered.

As the winter passed, a friend of mine came across a book called, *The Kingdom Assignment* (22). The book is based on the true story of a church pastor who provided his congregation with a unique challenge. He had a handful of one hundred-dollar bills and offered them to those present on that particular Sunday morning. There were three provisos. First, you had to acknowledge that this was God's money. Second, you had to take the money and do something of value to invest in "The Kingdom." Third, you agreed to come back to the church and tell the crowd what happened three months later. The book has several amazing stories. Some people raised thousands of dollars for charity, others bought books for poor people, some bought food for the homeless. I remember the story of a chiropractor who went downtown and barbecued hamburgers for the people living on the street. I was really inspired. Later that spring, that same friend challenged a bunch of us to do the assignment with fifty-dollar bills. I thought that it was a good idea but confess that I felt guilty about the wad of fifties I had stashed in my shaving kit.

Before we got rolling on the Kingdom Assignment, I got a call from the cycle shop that my bike was ready. It was about two months late, and I had been getting impatient. I remember driving to the shop with a wallet full of fifties. I looked at my bulging wallet as I walked from my car to the store. I felt a distinct sense of disappointment in myself. People had done such amazing things with just two fifties in the Kingdom Assignment, and I was doing something completely selfish, buying an expensive toy with *sooo* many fifties. I compartmentalized my guilt as walked in to pick up the bike.

The proprietor brought out my custom-made, brand new bike and I was perplexed. I had ordered a red bike, and this one was white. I asked the store owner what was going on, and he said he had changed the color! My feelings of guilt were now complicated by the weird vibe I was getting from the proprietor. I kept looking at the bike and noticed there was wear on the tires and a scratch on the side. I brought this to the attention of the owner, and he said that someone had test-ridden it for me and caused a little damage. My conscience was silently screaming at me and I decided that I wasn't going to take the bike. I asked the man for a refund of my $1000 deposit. I was expecting a fight, but he was quite agreeable. I had trouble believing the astonishing coincidence when he gave me twenty $50 bills. I now had sixty $50 bills in my wallet. All I could think about was the Kingdom Assignment.

I made my way home and pulled into the garage. I sat there in shock for several minutes and the significance of the whole thing struck me in a profound way. It seemed as if I had been deliberately steered away from the bike purchase and handed a chance to participate in the Kingdom Assignment with a stack of fifties. I got choked-up as I felt a sense of the supernatural at work.

The next time I saw my friend who issued the challenge to me, he told me he was starting a program to help inner-city kids go to summer camp. He was looking to raise some money and asked if I was able to help. I told him the story of the supernatural bike rebate and he was blown-away. This man, known for his crusty exterior and colorful language, actually began to weep. I ended up giving him half of the fifties for his inner-city kids. In the end we were both crying.

The Kingdom Assignment experience had been quite powerful for me. It seemed as though my friend and I had shared a supernatural "God moment." Nevertheless, as spring approached, I realized I had a first-world problem. Back when I thought I was getting a new bike, I had agreed to give my old bike to a friend's wife. After all, it had a late 80's retro-pink paint job. The woman had picked it up, and I found myself without wheels in the middle of triathlon season. The week after, I was driving home past a different cycle shop. They were advertising a sale and I popped into the store. It turned out that the young man working in the store was a provincial team triathlete and a friend of mine. He said he could get me a bike at half price. The bike he recommended was regularly priced at $3000, the precise value of the bike I had originally intended to purchase. He was also able to offer an additional "friends and family discount" of $500. I continued to feel the metaphysical at work. After paying for the bike, I still had a several fifties left in my wallet, fifties that would continue to have a supernatural fall-out.

Several weeks later, I was walking near the Mission over a lunch break. A man I recognized from Siloam approached me on the street, offering to sell me some trinkets for "a reasonable price." It was his gimmick for panhandling. I took a fifty from my wallet and told him that he didn't have to sell me anything. I tucked the fifty in his hands, trying not to let anyone on the street see. The big man dropped to his knees, grabbed me by the ankles and shouted, "Who are you and where are you from? Are you an angel?" I was mortified as there were people passing by on the street, enjoying a lunch-hour stroll. Some concerned citizens actually came over to make sure we were alright. I reassured them we were fine and helped the man to his feet. I walked with the homeless man for a while and we said goodbye. I was unnerved by the fellow's reaction and what seemed to be another amazing fifty. We were both a little shaken-up as we parted.

Months later, I was dropping off my nieces at a music studio a block away from Siloam where they took their piano lessons. After they got out of the car, a man approached my door and asked for money. I had one last fifty-dollar bill in my wallet and hoped I could engineer another memorable experience. I greeted the man and gave him the fifty. I must say I was disappointed when he simply grabbed it and ran. I thought all the fifties were supernatural. I went for a coffee while the girls were at their lessons and, when I returned, the man approached the car again. I thought he was returning to thank me and acknowledge the miraculous gift. I was sure he would say something amazing. When he knocked on the window, I eagerly rolled it down, but he had no recollection of our prior meeting and asked me again for money. I tried to remind him of the fifty dollars but he didn't have a clue. His face was blank and he simply moved on. It appeared that this Kingdom Assignment had come to its conclusion. It was quite a ride.

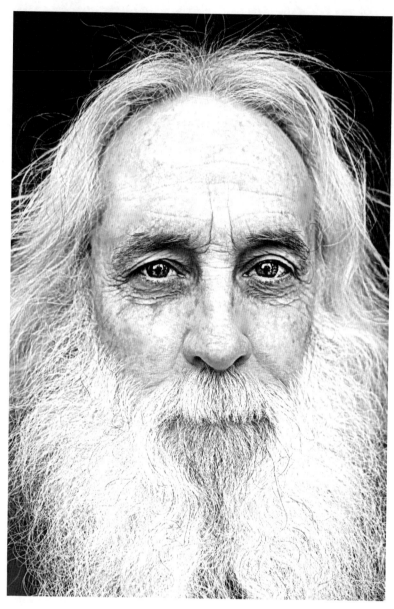

This photograph is taken with permission from Leah Denbok's work, *Nowhere to Call Home. Photographs and Stories of the Homeless. Volume One* or her website. It is not an image of any character referred to in this book. To see more of Leah's photography, visit ldenbokphotography.com.

LESSON 17:

Fear is a reaction,
courage is a decision.
—Sir Winston Churchill

*Success is not final. Failure is not fatal. It is the courage to
continue that counts.*
—Sir Winston Churchill

Many of the characters you meet at the Mission are so wonderfully unique you could suspect them of being actors. Are they sent from the medical college, simulated patients come to evaluate my clinical care? Joseph was one such inimitable character. He looked like he belonged at a university podium or on a cruise rather than at a homeless shelter. In his late 70's, Joseph was articulate and charismatic and moved with a fluid urgency seldom seen in men his age. His entrance complaint was simple. "Doc, I need you to clean out my f---ing ears." So, Joseph didn't speak like a professor.

Part of the medical evaluation process is reviewing a patient's past medical history, and when I asked Joseph if he had had any prior problems, he literally erupted. What followed was a torrent of criticism regarding the f---ing assholes he had encountered in the health care system. His medical journey had many ports of call.

Joseph started with the fact that he had terminal cancer. He had spent the last eight months dealing with medical malfeasance and had many stories to tell. F-bombs littered the room as he recounted a string of nightmarish medical scenarios. A nurse approaching him with "a needle big enough to tranquilize a horse", intending to "stick it where the sun don't shine" and who, when confronted, realized it was for the patient in the next bed. He told me of doctors pressuring him to go on a chemotherapy regimen who were offended and left the room when he had the gall to ask "what that shit might do to his healthy cells." He recounted firing many physicians for their arrogance and refusal to answer his questions. He expected some compassion in the medical process and, based on his testimony, he hadn't received it.

Despite his constellation of medical problems, Joseph did not have any pain and felt well. He didn't want his remaining days on earth to be dominated by "those assholes", nor did he want the burden of the side effects so common with chemotherapy. I told him I understood his decision and, if he did have terminal cancer, he looked amazingly well. I was determined not to be fired by him.

My task that day – to clean the wax out of Joseph's ears – is not up there with curing cancer on the hierarchy of medical interventions. Kate's only apparent flaw is that she seems to produce too much earwax and her external ear canals occasionally clog with it. As the physician on call for this emergency, I dutifully clean her ears with a large plastic syringe we have at home. Kate is somewhat critical of my technique, claiming that I hurt her ears, and she offers numerous tips on how to make the procedure better. I try to reassure her that I am a highly qualified medical professional with over 30 years of experience and that I am not hurting her ears. I remind her that my technique is based on ancient medical teachings handed down from Hippocrates himself. After all, a physician knows these things. I think Kate would fire me if she could, but I am generally the only available physician in the kitchen. For all you young spouses out there, never question your wife's pain threshold – it may lead to a test of yours.

The beauty of working at the Siloam clinic is that you can take your time with patients. You are there to practice medicine, but the motivation is different. As a volunteer, you are just there for the patients and the *business* of medicine is left completely out of the equation. Most of the clients are not in a hurry, not trying to get back to work or the kids to school. The less frenetic pace facilitates greater opportunity for simple human connection.

After what seemed like a half an hour of getting through Joseph's medical sojourn, I asked him if I could look in his ears. He jumped up on the bed with the grace of a young dancer. As I peered into his ear canal, he asked me if I could see through to the wall on the far side of the room, a common query from the comedic sort. I assured him that I could only see wax and that we should rinse it out.

I prepared Joe with a towel and kidney basin to catch the water that sprays out of the ear while trying to dislodge the wax. As we got started, he asked me if I had ever used Gin to wash out earwax. We had a good chuckle together at that. Dislodging ear wax is surprisingly gratifying. A deaf patient walks in and, with virtually no cost and few complications, hearing can be restored. The quantity of wax that can be syringed out is often quite amazing. Joe was duly impressed at the massive "piece of shit" that had been residing in his ear canal "rent free." We had another chuckle.

After we cleaned-up the splattered water from the earwax cleaning (Kate hates this part), I wanted to revisit Joseph's story of terminal cancer. He spoke in "riffs", staccato-like sentences that sounded rehearsed, detailing his many battles with the medical profession. It was very hard to get a word in, so I just sat back and listened. It was kind of fun watching a guy who looked like a well-travelled professor and sounded like the King of England, drop F-bombs on the medical establishment.

Amid the blue, somewhat pressured language was a story of bowel cancer with widespread intra-abdominal metastases. Joseph had been offered an extensive operation, chemotherapy and radiotherapy. He had refused them all. He was prepared to die. If he was afraid at this prospect, he did not show it. Joe's courage in light of his prognosis prompted me to re-examine my own fears of impairment, death and dying. How was he able to be so courageous when I was so afraid?

When I was back at the clinic the following week, Joe was my second patient of the morning. He greeted me like we were long-lost friends. He started talking in the waiting room and just kept on talking throughout our entire visit. He wanted a little tune-up on the right ear. The "Gin" line was used again, as were many of his riffs. What was clear was that I had established a connection with this unique fellow. Time did not allow a full unpacking of his 76-years of adventure but I am sure they were filled with amazing experiences. Joseph had terminal cancer. A single tear that he quickly brushed aside betrayed his emotional ambivalence with this reality. It saddened me to think of this delightful old man, alone at a homeless shelter, dying of cancer. It saddened me that he had a terminal illness and was forced to face down the medical system on his own. Yet, Joe had a fierce courage that was a central part of his unique character, far more courage than I had. Joseph reminded me of Winston Churchill's observation: fear is a reaction, courage a decision. Joe seemed to have made the right decision as he readied himself to die without heroic medical interventions. I have not seen him since.

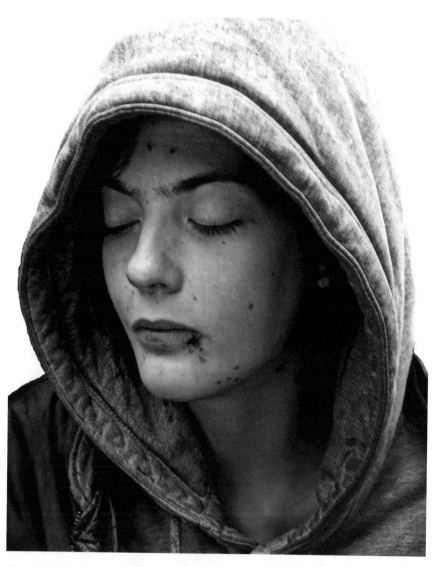

This photograph is taken with permission from Leah Denbok's work, *Nowhere to Call Home. Photographs and Stories of the Homeless. Volume One* or her website. It is not an image of any character referred to in this book. To see more of Leah's photography, visit ldenbokphotography.com.

LESSON 18: Pain and suffering are the soil of strength and courage.

—Lurlene McDaniel

Although the world is full of suffering, it is also full of the overcoming of it.
—Helen Keller

Before clinic one morning, I was asked to see Kim, a Siloam volunteer who needed some help with her medication. Angelika informed me that her doctor was away and she hoped I could do her a favor. Kim was a young Indigenous woman, well-groomed and well-dressed. She was soft-spoken with a very somber affect. She needed some Effexor, an anti-depressant. She had run out, and her family doctor was out of town. Given that she was a volunteer and that Effexor is not an abused drug, this seemed like a straightforward request. I asked her how long she had been on the medication and she responded that it had only been three weeks. When I asked her what had prompted the need for the anti-depressants, she rolled up her sleeves and showed me fresh cut marks on her arms. They were still bleeding. Before I could ask her anything about the cuts, she began to tell me of her remarkably painful journey through life.

Kim had been abandoned by her birth mother at the age of two. She had lived most of her life in Hamilton, in foster care, 13 families by her estimation. She had been physically and sexually abused by several of the foster parents. After years searching for her birth family, she had managed to find her uncle – her mom's brother – and moved back to Winnipeg to live with him. This had not turned out well. She learned that her mother was dead, a probable victim in the missing and murdered Indigenous women cohort. Her uncle's spouse had a daughter from a previous relationship, and that young woman had just been found dead in a McDonald's bathroom, another victim of the opioid crisis having overdosed on methadone. The surviving spouse was now on suicide watch at a hospital in the city, and Kim was concerned that her uncle was also going to kill himself. She sat in the examining room contemplating the deaths that had happened, the ones possibly to come, and her own self-injurious behavior.

Even as Kim was thinking of harming herself, she was wrestling with her mortality. Before she could finish describing her family situation, she opened her shirt and showed me a foot-long scar over her breast bone. She had a major cardiac defect that had required one operation and would need another within the year. She was on multiple cardiac medications and blood thinners, which explained why her slash marks were still oozing with blood. I couldn't imagine how a woman in her twenties could have suffered more.

Kim was remarkably forthcoming about her suicidal thoughts. She told me she had a plan: she was going to hang herself. She didn't think she could face any more tragedy. I explained to her that when someone reveals these thoughts, my response has to be to protect the patient from themselves, often by having them urgently assessed at the hospital, if not apprehended by the police. She responded that she didn't intend to kill herself today, because she had to help her uncle make funeral arrangements for her step-sister. We spent a great deal of time discussing our next steps. I shared with Kim my familiarity with suicide and its impact on a family through the story of my brother's death. I think that helped build some trust between us. I stated the obvious, that her path through life had been full of more suffering than perhaps any other I had encountered in my career. I tried to convey to her that I understood a bit of where she was. She seemed to understand that suicide just passes pain from one person to another.

I was very concerned at the prospect of Kim going anywhere other than straight to the hospital. We discussed the idea of a suicide contract, that she would vow not to harm herself and, if she felt she couldn't honor her pledge, that she would attend an emergency room for help. Kim appeared to be honest with me and said that she would not harm herself in the coming days. She was hoping to support her uncle through the funeral arrangements and the grief he was enduring. She seemed very intent on doing something good, something positive.

I felt that familiar apprehension that comes when a patient with major problems is about to leave your care. Would she harm herself more seriously today? Should I call the police? I asked Kim if I could speak with Angelika about her situation. She agreed and Angelika and I went through the options for this poor woman. Angelika was very helpful in our deliberations. She knew Kim and believed that she really wanted to help her uncle and was convinced that she would not do any more harm to herself that day. We hoped she would be okay, persevering under the mountain of suffering on her shoulders. It struck me how strong she was in the eye of this storm. Kim wasn't trying to draw sympathy. She wasn't being melodramatic. The contradiction between her horrible past and her strong desire to contribute something of value to her uncle was very inspiring. Kim was a living example that suffering produces endurance, and endurance produces character, and character produces hope. (23) Hope allows us to continue to walk in the tempest. Kim was doing just that.

At a subsequent shift at the clinic, I inquired how Kim was doing. Angelika informed me that she was working through her troubles and looking a bit better. Kim reinforced for us the truth of Hellen Keller's words, herself no stranger to difficulty – the world is full of suffering, but it is also full of the overcoming of it.

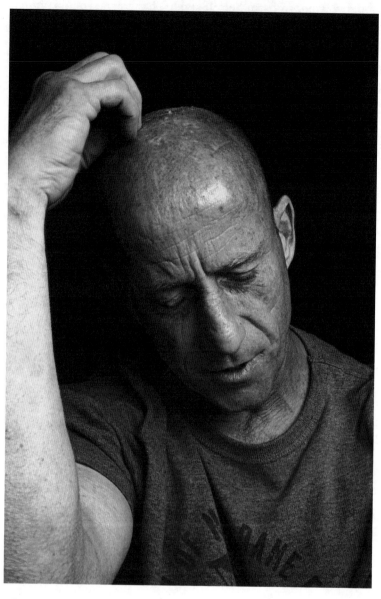

This photograph is taken with permission from Leah Denbok's work, *Nowhere to Call Home. Photographs and Stories of the Homeless. Volume One* or her website. It is not an image of any character referred to in this book. To see more of Leah's photography, visit ldenbokphotography.com.

LESSON 19: Success is knowing your purpose, appropriating your gifts, and sowing seeds that benefit others.

—Ralph Mueller

See one, do one, teach one.
—Medical training principle

There is a terrifying saying in medical education: *See one, do one, teach one.* The principle is that after you see a procedure done once, you are capable of performing it, and then, after performing it, you are able to teach someone else. My most powerful memory of this occurred in my fourth year of medical school, on the wards during a surgical rotation. A frail, elderly woman had fluid in her chest cavity known as a pleural effusion. This fluid needs to be analyzed to determine its cause and must be aspirated via a large bore syringe inserted directly into the thorax of the patient. This particular woman seemed so vulnerable and was very short of breath. My supervising resident asked me if I had ever seen the procedure, known as a thoracentesis. I had not, so my resident demonstrated the technique, and then said "You'll do the next one."

I was prone to fainting during medical school. It happened probably 20 times. My most embarrassing faint was when I observed my first circumcision. Surrounded by a group of young moms in a neonatal ward, we were practicing our examinations of newborns, when a kindly old obstetrician came in. He asked me if I had ever seen a circumcision and offered me the chance to assist. I thought this would be a valuable experience, and joined the doctor at the young lad's crib. The last thing I remember was our startled little patient's wailing as the forceps clamped down on his foreskin.

As I regained consciousness, I became aware that they had dumped me into a rocking chair, draped me in a bright yellow hospital gown, and nestled a baby doll in my arms. A photograph of this humiliating scene remained on the "Proud Moms" bulletin board for the remainder of the rotation. That was just one reason I didn't pursue obstetrics.

Cut back to the thoracentesis. As I witnessed the thick fluid being drawn out of the patient's chest into a massive syringe, I started to feel queasy. The resident recognized my facial pallor and sweaty brow, and suggested I sit down with my head between my knees. She shared with me that she too had been a fainter in medical school, but was now able to train as a surgeon, free of the problem. She helped me realize that I had to focus on the task at hand, not just empathize with the suffering patient. Ultimately, completing the task would help the patient and that was the goal. I was able to perform the next thoracentesis on our frail patient when the effusion re-accumulated. Her breathing was easier afterward, and I didn't faint. I think that was when my fainting stopped. The resident's kindness to me gave me my first glimpse into the world of being a good medical educator.

One of my favorite things to do at Siloam is to work with aspiring doctors. The medical problems at the Mission are so diverse and different from what you would see in a standard family practice setting. As a result, the experience provides a unique opportunity for learners. I also hope that the students will feel the joy that can be found in serving the homeless people and learn some lessons that only they can teach. I have mentioned Rachel, my niece, who has probably been my most faithful student. My son has spent a few days with me. I have had two physicians from Egypt work alongside me at Siloam, as well as a young beefcake ex-bartender who was doing his training in the United States. His good looks seemed to bring out a special group of volunteers to help around the clinic, mostly young women.

One particular Friday, I was working with another young pre-med student, Andrew. My relationship with Andrew is a classic example of the "two degrees of separation" one finds in Winnipeg. Everyone knows everyone. Both of Andrew's parents are doctors and both were my classmates in medical school. Early in my career, I worked with Andrew's paternal grandparents, both physicians. His grandfather was one of the city's most respected surgeons and his grandmother, a psychiatrist, practiced well into her eighties. Andrew also worked at a summer camp with my daughter and son. Andrew is an exceptional young man – brilliant, witty, articulate and passionate, a national champion debater. I love the way he engages with patients when I leave the room. He treats them with respect and genuine interest.

Our first patient of the day was a man named Morris, who we were asked to see by Chris, the chiropractor who volunteers at the Mission on Thursday evenings. Chris had seen Morris the night before and was concerned he might have an ominous spinal condition known as cauda equina syndrome. The condition involves pressure on the nerves of the cauda equina or "horse's tail." This group of nerves begins at the termination of the spinal cord at the first lumbar vertebra. The nerves then course through the spinal canal, responsible for the transmission of motor and sensory function to the legs, as well as the muscles that control the bladder and bowel sphincters. Cauda equina syndrome, usually caused by a massive disc herniation and the pressure exerted on the nerves, can lead to paralysis of the legs as well as permanent problems with urinary and fecal incontinence. As such, it constitutes a medical emergency that requires urgent surgical decompression. It is one of a handful of "red flag" conditions that can affect the lumbar spine.

Morris was a black man in his late thirties. He was a new Canadian, having emigrated from Central Africa about a year before. Refugees are a growing demographic in homeless shelters, and so we see many newcomers to Canada at Siloam. Morris was bright-eyed and pleasant. I explained to him that the chiropractor had left me a note outlining his concern about possible cauda equina problems. Morris wanted to know what this meant and why it was such a big deal. I reviewed the pathophysiology of the condition for both Morris and Andrew, and then asked the patient how all this had started. That's when things got interesting.

Morris told us that he lived in his own 7-bedroom home and had been doing some renovations on its turn-of-the-century structure. He claimed that, three months prior to seeing us, he had lifted up a door frame and supported over 1000 pounds. He had felt a sudden intense pain in his back and trouble with both legs. He told us he had been in and out of the hospital ever since. He had developed infections of both of his kidneys as well as swelling in his legs. There was concern that he had blood clots, and he had been put on blood thinners for a short period of time. The story then became even more bizarre when he told us it had been discovered that he had 400% of the usual amount of testosterone in his system. He started doing body-builder poses, showing off his impressive biceps. I told him I wasn't expecting a gun show and didn't have my holster. We all chuckled.

Morris went on to tell us that he was a millionaire and had retired in Africa while in his thirties and had come to Canada for adventure. He had run a marathon in under two hours and thirty minutes, a time, even most elite runners, would never be able to achieve. He denied that he was staying at the Mission, explaining that he was just visiting someone. I began to see a familiar pattern at play. I suspected that Morris was manic. It can be difficult to elucidate prior mental illness in a person who does not want to disclose any past diagnoses or treatment. Yet, the pressured speech, the grandiose claims and the tangential thinking all convinced me that Morris was bipolar. He still needed to be evaluated for the potential cauda equina syndrome, and this would complicate matters.

The assessment for cauda equina syndrome requires a careful neurological examination, including documentation of the sensation in the perineal area between the scrotum and anus. A rectal examination is also required to ensure that the muscles that control bowel function are intact. I wanted to preserve Morris' dignity, so I suggested Andrew could leave the room if he felt uncomfortable having a learner present. Morris was happy to help in the education process and proceeded to undress and wanted us to note his rather impressive abdominal six-pack. I acknowledged that his musculature was impressive but was also concerned that his legs were quite swollen. He assured me that the swelling had been present since that first trip to the hospital three months ago and had been evaluated with ultrasounds, ruling out blood clots in his legs. Andrew was seeing some real pathology and, thankfully, he was not a fainter. As I performed his rectal examination, I asked Morris to contract his anal sphincter, and was thankful that he demonstrated normal tone, as well as normal sensation in the entire region. This is an important sign indicating normal nerve function of the cauda equina. It was reassuring. Morris continued his string of hyperbolic observations after we finished, boasting that he could have crushed my finger by contracting "a thousand times harder." He quipped that he refrained from hurting me as he didn't want to become known as "the asshole that hurt the doc." We all chuckled.

The good news was that Morris did not have any of the worrisome features of cauda equina syndrome, but he did have a sore back and swollen legs and we had to try to help him. I also wanted to see if he had any insight into his potential psychiatric condition. I asked about prior medications, hospitalizations and doctors, but he gave us nothing. He did tell us that he had an appointment with an old friend, the city's best spine surgeon, in just three days. His buddy, the surgeon, had looked after him in the past. Morris would not stop talking and regaled us with one story after another, each slightly more incredible than the last. He talked so long that Angelika actually had to summon me out of the examination room to punctuate the visit, as the other patients were starting to complain.

As we ended the visit, Morris asked me to prescribe him some morphine. I had actually been waiting for this. He had not been able to get to the doctor who usually provided this medication for him. We told Morris that we do not prescribe opioids at the Mission clinic. Fears of drug diversion and facilitating substance abuse are two of the key reasons. Patients receiving opioids have been mugged in the past, having their drugs stolen as they leave the clinic. Also, this class of drugs is generally not indicated for chronic, non-malignant pain. They simply don't work for most people. Opioids are effective for the short-term management of acute pain syndromes such as trauma or post-surgical cases. They are also a major plank in the management of palliative care patients, able to ease the pain of the dying. However, many management guidelines recommend caution in using opioids in the treatment of conditions like back pain. Morris did not challenge our position and simply responded, "It doesn't hurt to ask."

The visit with Morris was a great learning opportunity for Andrew. Our patient had taught him about an important medical condition and added several pearls about physical examination. Morris had demonstrated that psychological filters and psychosocial issues affect the presentation of physical problems.

After Morris left, I asked what Andrew thought of our patient. I wanted to see if he had realized that Morris was probably bipolar. Andrew was interested in the leg edema, and the back pain but made no mention of his other behavior. I recapped that our patient was attending a homeless shelter but was a retired 30-year old millionaire who owned a 7-bedroom house, ran a world-class marathon, had four times the average amount of male testosterone, couldn't stop talking and had the world's strongest asshole. Andrew started to smile and acknowledged that our patient had some fairly grandiose thoughts. The visit highlighted the difficulty of seeing someone at the point in their illness trajectory where they just seem unusual, not psychiatrically ill. Morris was not a threat to himself at that moment. He was not a threat to others. I suspected he was headed down a tough road, but he either didn't want to acknowledge it or lacked the insight to realize it.

We had another bipolar patient that morning, a sixty-five-year old man with an outlandish wig of long, straight, red hair. He reminded me of a "Spice Girl." He was agitated and seemed angry with us, until he realized that Andrew had met him over the weekend, serving him coffee at Siloam's drop-in center. Andrew had been volunteering there, despite being in full time university studies and trying to get into medicine. With a more conciliatory attitude, our mop-topped patient began to chatter on with Andrew and was remarkably tangential. He talked about everything, except why he wanted to see the doctor. I asked him several times how we could help him but he got angry every time I interrupted him. Ironically, he said that he wanted to see a psychiatrist to deal with his anger issues.

We agreed to refer him to a community-based psychiatrist. It took a half an hour to get to this result.

Andrew and I chatted about the morning's patients as we ended our shift. He told me that he wanted to work as a rural family doctor. He was volunteering at the Mission to learn something about medicine as well as to just hang out, serving people. He seemed to have a heart for those who were struggling and genuinely cared about the people who were homeless. Andrew acknowledged that the process of trying to get into medicine was a daunting one. Rachel and my son were both in their first year of medicine, so I knew he was right. I was reminded of the difficulties on my own path to becoming a physician. The morning with Andrew reminded me of the definition of success one of my friends has coined: know your purpose, appropriate your gifts and sow seeds that benefit others. Using this template, Andrew was already a success.

The story of Morris had a very sad epilogue. We finally got a packet of his medical records from our regional health authority. His complaints of back pain, leg swelling and trouble walking had been present for at least four months. He had close to thirty visits to emergency rooms in our city, literally going in every other day with similar complaints. He was labeled as "drug-seeking and manipulative" and considered to have a narcissistic personality disorder. His grandiose claims were noted by some of the physicians, but there had been no psychiatric consultation. The MRI of his spine did not show any worrisome features. All of the records noted his long-term, high-dose morphine use. With the benefit of hindsight, you could see his inevitable descent into an opioid-induced psychosis.

I asked Angelika if we could locate Morris and bring him back to the clinic to discuss these matters and try to convince him to get some psychiatric care. She told me that Morris had continued to deteriorate emotionally. He had become increasingly agitated and threatened to re-visit the Mission with a knife and kill all the staff. I shared this information with Andrew. Dozens of interactions with the medical system had failed to prevent his slide into the abyss. We silently mourned the news of this tragic end. Morris's superhuman strength was no match for the relentless duo of mental illness and substance abuse that keep filling up our streets.

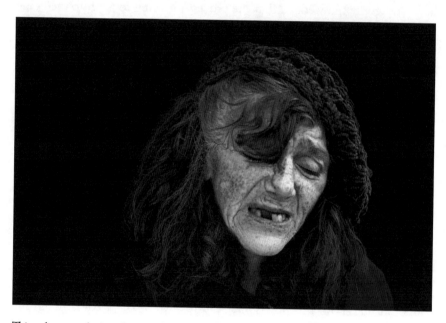

This photograph is taken with permission from Leah Denbok's work, *Nowhere to Call Home. Photographs and Stories of the Homeless. Volume One* or her website. It is not an image of any character referred to in this book. To see more of Leah's photography, visit ldenbokphotography.com.

LESSON 20 :

Listen to people. Hearing someone's burden can lighten it.

Wherever the art of medicine is loved, there is also a love of humanity.
—Hippocrates

Laugh with your happy friends when they're happy; share tears when they're down. Get along with each other; don't be stuck-up. Make friends with nobodies; don't be the great somebody.
—Romans 12, The Message

Have you ever felt that someone really heard what you had to say? Really listened? Doctors are often criticized for not listening to their patients. Statistics say that doctors typically interrupt their patients within the first 30 seconds of the patient's story. Yikes.

I have had the great blessing of being listened to. For the last twenty years, five men and I meet every Friday morning at 7 am. We come together to help each other walk as authentic followers of Jesus. This group has been one of the greatest sources of help, healing and wise counsel in my life. We call it our accountability group. We show up every Friday with no agenda and no preparation, have a prayer, and someone poses the simple question: OK, who's got stuff? What flows from this query is an hour and a half of candid conversation about all the important aspects of our lives. We have been through births and deaths, marriage failures and successes, business challenges as well as many victories. We have supported each other despite moral failure, stupidity, duplicity and hubris. We have also shared lots of laughs and joy. We have relied on the Spirit to lead us into truth and make us aware of each other's problems. These five strong men have provided me with compassion, guidance, kindness, wisdom, forgiveness, correction, hope and love. The most important thing they do is listen.

I was working with Andrew on a cold and blustery January morning. Our first patient of the day was another poor soul whose life had been shattered by bipolar disorder. Gladys was a Metis woman in her late 60's, new to the Mission. She had seen the nurse the day before but would not disclose her troubled psychiatric past. Appropriately, the nurse was concerned about her unusual behavior and asked her to see me. The staff were worried about the possibility of a new psychotic episode, toxic delirium, or organic brain disease.

As soon as we settled in the examination room, Gladys unraveled the mystery and calmly explained that she had had bipolar disorder since youth and was on Valproic acid, a mood stabilizer. She had an excellent psychiatrist in the city who was modifying her medical regimen and seeing her on a regular basis. For some reason, she thought the clinic nurse was part of the vast conspiracy out to get her. I was relieved that we wouldn't have to go on a medical sleuthing expedition to account for her behavior. She actually seemed quite calm, well-oriented to her surroundings and to have good insight into her psychiatric condition. She was a very likeable person. That made it all the more difficult to see her carrying two heavy winter coats and a large duffle bag, full of all her worldly goods. She could barely manage to haul it down the short corridor of the clinic. How did she manage to cope on the frigid streets in January? I could hardly imagine.

We asked Gladys if she was staying at the Mission and she informed us she had been there for three weeks. We asked what had happened to account for her stay at Siloam, and that was when her incredible story of trouble tumbled out. She had been living at a group home and one of the tenants there had tried to assault her. She fled from the apartment and headed to another shelter in the city's core area. She said that, as she was being escorted to her room, the shelter attendant stopped the elevator and also assaulted her. She escaped and made her way to Siloam where she finally felt safe.

Gladys talked about being estranged from her husband and all of her children. She was also alienated from her family of origin, who she described as intolerant and judgmental. I'm sure they would have a different perspective, given the many challenges of living with sufferers of bipolar disorder. She recounted her toxic relationship with her father and alleged that he had surreptitiously poisoned her over the years. Gladys blamed her father's pharmaceutical meddling for her mental illness. She suspected that he was still trying to harm her with strange and illicit chemicals. From her account, it was difficult to distinguish truth from paranoid delusion. Gladys' speech intensified as she told us of all the people who had harmed her, dating back to her adolescence. Again, these were cited as the causes of her mental illness. It was so hard to sort out cause and effect, to know whether the injuries were real or imagined. To Gladys, though, those were distinctions without a difference. Her pain was the same and it was real.

It was profoundly sad to think of this vulnerable older woman being hurt and living on the street. Gladys needed some more of her medications, as she had left them behind during her escape. We organized the appropriate prescriptions for her, and as I was typing up her documents, Andrew continued to engage her in conversation. More incredible details of her life emerged. She told stories of exotic travels, but all of her journeys seemed to end in tragedy. She was completely at ease with Andrew and they talked for quite awhile. We didn't *do* anything in the traditional biomedical model. Most of all we listened. At the end of our visit, she remarked how good it was to talk and how safe she felt at Siloam. She felt that her burden was a little lighter.

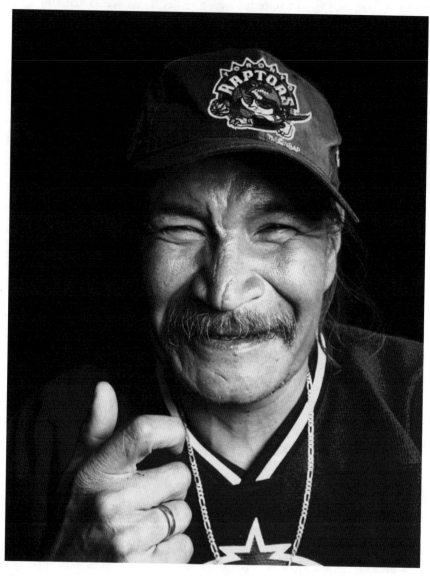

This photograph is taken with permission from Leah Denbok's work, *Nowhere to Call Home. Photographs and Stories of the Homeless. Volume One* or her website. It is not an image of any character referred to in this book. To see more of Leah's photography, visit ldenbokphotography.com.

Our last patient of the morning was a large Inuit man. Nathan probably weighed 250 pounds. His right arm was very muscular, covered with tattoos and I recognized some symbols of gang affiliation. His left arm was similarly adorned with tattoos, but considerably smaller and deformed. He had told the triage person that he wanted help with chronic pain, and I worried that he would be agitated if I refused to provide him with opiate analgesics. I was a little apprehensive at the outset of our visit, thankful that Andrew was with me.

Nathan was in his early thirties and had a really bad arm. He told us his arm had been mangled in an industrial accident in the Northwest Territories, the limb caught in a snow-throwing auger. He had undergone several surgical procedures that had not been very helpful. He had just moved to Winnipeg from Yellowknife and was out of all of his pain medication. He informed us that he was using Percocet, an opioid analgesic, and gabapentin. I told Nathan that I would not be able to prescribe him the Percocet as clinic policy prohibited it. I was braced for an angry response but he answered meekly that he understood, but he really hoped we could prescribe the gabapentin. He said it really helped him with his nerves.

Gabapentin is a medicine originally designed to help people with epilepsy. It is effective in the prevention of seizures. Over the last 15 years, it has also become a staple in the management of chronic neuropathic pain. When a nerve is damaged, it can emit continual pain impulses that can be difficult to eradicate. Gabapentin seems to be effective in this context. It has the added advantage of not being addictive and seems to be diverted less than the opiates and benzodiazepines. I asked Nathan if his nerve had been damaged in the surgery when it became clear that the *nerves* he referred to were his emotions. In a quavering voice, that giant of a man told us of the death of his wife. In the most tender reflection, he told us she was another victim of the fentanyl epidemic. He stared off into space as he recalled the difficulty of finding her lifeless body. He had never recovered from the experience. Nathan's eyes were moist as he described adopting his spouse's children nine years ago. Those relationships had not turned out well.

Nathan's recent move into Winnipeg had been prompted by another tragedy related to the opioid crisis. His cousin had just died from an overdose of methadone, a synthetic opioid used to treat people addicted to this class of drugs. The theory goes that methadone mitigates the craving of opioids without getting people high. It also staves off the pain of withdrawal. One complication with methadone is that it is usually administered on a daily basis – just a small volume of liquid – to prevent diversion and overdose. Patients are required to attend the methadone clinic daily to get their medication but may be given three doses on a Friday to "carry-over" through the weekend. Nathan's cousin took his three doses home and drank them all at once. Because methadone doesn't give the patient a recognizable high, the addict may be driven to take more, searching for relief that never comes. Methadone can have a very deleterious effect on the heart's electrical conduction, leading to a particularly lethal heart rhythm. Nathan's cousin had died as a result of this complication, and again, Nathan had discovered the lifeless body. He had left the North looking for respite from the tragedies "on the other side of the wall."

Nathan was clearly shaken-up. This man, built like a bull, was vulnerable and frightened. His loved ones had been stolen by the opioid epidemic. It boggled our minds how this scourge had found its way even to a remote corner of Canada's Northwest Territories, only a couple of hundred miles from the Arctic circle. Again, as I prepared Nathan's prescription for gabapentin on the electronic medical record, Andrew engaged him in conversation. He was able to get Nathan to laugh a few times through his tears. It was clear Nathan was in pain and, more than any medication, he needed someone to listen to his story. The three of us seemed to make a quick connection, a small port in a complicated storm. Nathan was very thankful for his time with us. As I gave him his prescription, he looked us both in the eye and shook our hands with considerable vigor with his powerful right arm. He said he felt as if his burden had lightened. What more could we ask for?

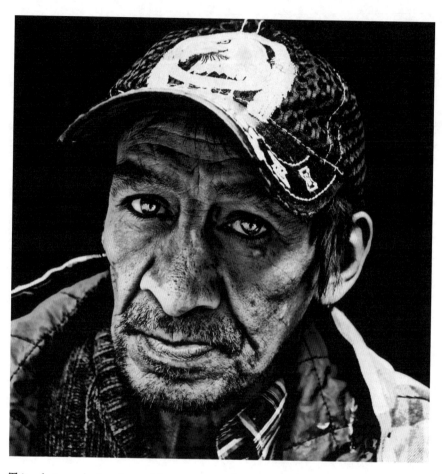

This photograph is taken with permission from Leah Denbok's work, *Nowhere to Call Home. Photographs and Stories of the Homeless. Volume One* or her website. It is not an image of any character referred to in this book. To see more of Leah's photography, visit ldenbokphotography.com.

LESSON 21:

Hardships often prepare people for an extraordinary destiny.
—CS Lewis

Give me knowledge so I can have kindness for all.
—wisdom saying of Plains Indians

Why are you homeless? What happened to you? I suspect these questions reflect affluent arrogance, what might be referred to in the modern vernacular as white privilege. Why are you on the street? Something must have gone wrong to account for your situation. Everybody is supposed to have a home, right? When I meet a person at the homeless Mission who seems kind, intelligent and well-spoken, I feel like I need to know what happened to push them to the streets. Part of the medical interview process involves the exploration of a person's social and family history with questions about where you live. I often ask patients if they are staying at Siloam, and if so, for how long. The question is straightforward, and people give immediate answers. On occasion, I will ask patients *why* they are at the Mission. Invariably, the patients struggle with the response. I suspect that the answers are very complicated.

There is a story in Leah Denbok's book, *Nowhere to Call Home. Photographs and Stories of the Homeless. Volume One,* where she describes meeting a homeless man whose story reflects this reality. (24) Ronny was on the street, having been kicked to the curb by several tragedies in his life. The beginning of his journey was when his 6-year old daughter died from cancer. Soon after, his wife took her own life. Ronny turned to substance use to cope with the pain and found himself with a $500-a-week habit. He was living paycheck to paycheck, when he literally found himself locked out of his home. Why was he homeless? There was no simple answer. A judgmental person would say the reason was alcohol, whereas a merciful person would say the reason was childhood cancer. I encountered a man at the Mission who answered my *why* question with a response that challenged how I thought about homelessness.

Percival was an Indigenous man in his late sixties. He was a stereotypical little old man, weighing at most 120 pounds. He had regal features with high cheek bones and a calm, unflappable manner. Percival used a walker to get around, as he had a cancerous lesion in his right hip region. This was supposed to have been surgically removed, but he missed his appointment and had not gotten a make-up date. He also suffered from a neurological disorder that affected his legs and this caused additional difficulty walking. Percival had a sleep disturbance and was having regular episodes of lightheadedness that seemed to be due to low blood pressure. At a recent trip to the hospital, it was also determined that he might have cancer affecting his brain, as well as a blood clot affecting his arm. After a previous visit, the Mission clinic had arranged to have the results of the hospital tests sent over, and then had tried to contact Percival to organize appropriate follow-up. It was about three weeks before he returned to the Mission and I was able discuss his test results with him.

I was happy to see Percival again. We had made a good connection several months earlier when he first started noticing the weakness and lightheadedness. I told him I was worried he was falling through the cracks of our medical system. This simple statement seemed to resonate with him; I think he viewed me as an ally after that. I told him that we had been trying to find him and asked where he had been. Percival responded, "I was on the street." This was particularly astonishing because we had just been through a cold snap that had enveloped most of North America. Wind chill values below -40 C had been recorded for several days in a row. I couldn't fathom how this delicate-looking, older man could have navigated the frigid streets of Winnipeg overnight with his walker, not to mention all of his physical impairments. I then asked the question that so many homeless patients seem to struggle with: "*Why* were you sleeping on the street?" Percival's incredible response was: "It's my *destiny*."

I didn't know if he was poking fun at me, but as I sat in stunned silence, he explained his perspective. Percival was an elder in his reserve community and had a responsibility to look after his people. He said that many of his people were living on the street around the Mission, so that was where he had to serve them. As he understood it, his destiny was shepherding his people on the streets of Winnipeg, despite temperatures colder than Mars. I marveled at his strength. I said how much I admired his tenacity, and he shrugged it off saying that he was only using "his gift." I asked what gift he was referring to and he became emotional. Through his tears, Percival recounted a visit from a *spirit guide* who had advised him of his sacred responsibilities. His gifts were not physical, but ones of knowledge, eloquence and resilience. His responsibility was to help his people wherever they were. His gifts of a sound mind and the ability to articulate the truths of Indigenous heritage to his people weighed heavily on him. Percival was serious about the stewardship of his gift.

Percival's perspective challenged many of the prejudices I held in my heart about the homeless. I believed that there must be something wrong with you if you were on the street. A mistake had been made, an error committed, a lapse in judgment, a moral failing. But Percival went willingly to the street to serve his people and his Creator, a noble calling. I reflected back on my walk in to the clinic that morning. Some of the neighboring buildings were being demolished and, because the normal parking lot beside the Mission was barricaded up, I had to detour through a longer route. I had thought smugly of how tough I was, roughing it, as I walked through the valley of the shadow of the mean streets in the frigid temperatures. Then I considered Percival. How humbling.

Percival wanted to know if the test results allowed us to determine how long he had left. I informed him that additional testing was required to define the nature of the brain tumor, but that the original impression was that the tumor was benign. I reassured him that most of the investigations looked good and that there were no imminent threats to his life. He smiled through his tears and then shared that his spirit guide had told him he had two years left to accomplish his tasks. Percival was not worried about the end; he just wanted to fulfill his mission: to serve his people. It was, after all, his destiny.

CLOSING THOUGHTS

A friend of mine was asked to give a talk about where people meet God. The 72-year old man reflected on an experience he had hiking the Great Divide trail that straddles the Rocky Mountains in Western North America. He was awestruck by the multitude of stars that met his gaze one perfectly clear night, far from the urban sprawl. He contemplated how insignificant he was in the infinite universe, and yet how marvelously complex . . . all ten trillion cells of his body working together in miraculous interdependence. In that moment, he felt he had met God. Infinity, simplicity, complexity, stillness, wonder, unity. It was a transcendent moment for him.

Where do you meet God? Have you ever considered the question? I have previously reflected on the faith tradition I follow – that, when we serve people in need, we serve God himself. The teachings of Jesus on the imperative of helping the needy is the central foundation of this book. Permit me to review it one last time.

Jesus provides his followers with a profound motivation to assist those who are struggling:

> *Then the King will say to those on his right, 'Enter, you who are blessed by my Father! Take what's coming to you in this kingdom. It's been ready for you since the world's foundation. And here's why:*
> *I was hungry and you fed me,*
> *I was thirsty and you gave me a drink,*
> *I was homeless and you gave me a room,*

I was shivering and you gave me clothes,
I was sick and you stopped to visit,
I was in prison and you came to me.'
"Then those 'sheep' are going to say, 'Master, what are you
talking about? When did we ever see you hungry and feed you,
thirsty and give you a drink? And when did we ever see you
sick or in prison and come to you?' Then the King will say, 'I'm
telling the solemn truth: Whenever you did one of these things
to someone overlooked or ignored, that was me—you did it
to me.'
Matthew 25, The Message (10)

Where do we meet God? This passage explains that whenever we serve those in need, we actually meet God there and then. Thirsty, hungry, homeless, sick, shivering, overlooked, ignored and in prison. Does anything sound more like the people attending a shelter for street people in Winnipeg? Those words sound as if they were written specifically about Siloam Mission, and countless other homeless shelters throughout the world. Apparently, the plight of homelessness existed 2,000 years ago. Apparently, Jesus wanted something done about it. And apparently, I can meet Him while I do something about it.

A friend recently told me of a weekend his family spent with a young girl fleeing from foster care. She was suicidal, damaged by multiple rapes at the hand of her foster father. She met my friend's family at a camp the prior summer. The young girl knew she could trust this family and that they would help her. The girl approached my friend's daughter in a time of great suffering. She had been working the streets and was in trouble with her pimp. After being taken in by my friend's family, given shelter and love, she said the exact words that Sam, the blind man, had uttered: "I have never been treated with such kindness." Their kindness opened a heart shut by violence, a mind closed by pain, and a spirit shut by condemnation. They demonstrated that love is an action, not an emotion. When they took in this young woman, they met God.

When people come to serve at missions like Siloam and are trying to help a homeless person, they are actually meeting Jesus there. That is the point of His story. Jesus said the greatest commandment is to love God with everything you have – your heart, mind, soul and strength – and the second, to love your neighbor as you love yourself. Jesus explained that a neighbor is not someone just like us. In fact, loving your neighbor, as Jesus saw it, meant bridging traditional "we-they" divides to serve those different from us, those far outside our circle of family and friends.

One meets people at a homeless shelter who are extremely vulnerable and in great need. The suffering faced by those on the street can seem insurmountable. The problems are so complicated and multi-dimensional that we are tempted to give up and move on. Some choose not to think about them at all. Yet, we need to remind ourselves and each other that a single act of mercy can make a difference in a person's life.

You will encounter incredibly memorable characters at a shelter. While many of the homeless seem stuck in a quagmire of struggles with health and addiction and are profoundly sad, you will also meet people who manifest inexplicable joy. With powerful testimonies of overcoming, these people remind us of our own weakness and of our God who meets us in that weakness. As I watch the people in the Mission offer up kindness, mercy and hope through their own vulnerability, I see the joy that can be found in serving others.

I believe you *can* meet God on a majestic hiking trail in the Rocky Mountains or on a black diamond ski run. But Jesus promises that I *will* meet God when I work at a homeless shelter because He is there, waiting patiently to see that the overlooked and ignored are being served. And because of that, I know there will be wisdom there too.

WORDS OF THANKS

I would like to thank some of the people who helped along this journey. The first is Carrie Enns, the original director of the Saul Sair Health Care Centre. She was a driving force to help the homeless, full of passion and grace. Vicki Olatundun, my second boss at Siloam, was likewise a force of nature, supplementing the clinic's resources with her charm and strength. Her training as a lawyer helped her to be a strong and forceful advocate for the homeless. She was also a lot of fun (and a great singer). Thank you to Angelika Fletcher, our current director, who is a source of kindness and unflappable support. She encouraged me in the writing of this book by reading it to her blind husband and telling me they had shared a tear and a laugh as they remembered our patients. I also want to thank all the other faithful health care providers who work at Siloam. Your silent service speaks volumes about your character.

Heartfelt thanks to my sister, Chris. I sent her an early draft of this manuscript and she surprised me by saying this had to go somewhere. She has read through multiple iterations, and her editorial wisdom and affection have been much appreciated. My friend, Professor Jane Lothian, also reviewed the original manuscript. She has co-authored a Sociology textbook and I wanted to get her thoughts on the project. She wept as we discussed some of the characters described in the book. Jane's encouragement provided impetus to continue on my writing journey. My sister, Lynn, also reviewed the book and provided insightful suggestions and encouragement.

I would like to thank my wife, Kate. She has been very patient with this project. It is definitely outside of her comfort zone. She spent hours going through the manuscript and used her highly-developed editorial skills to improve it immeasurably. I love her and am thankful for her. She provided substantial literary expertise and made the book much easier to read.

I need to thank all of the homeless people who have allowed me into their lives. The sacred moments of human connection I have shared with these people continue to shape who I am. The strength and resilience of these people are something to behold. By telling their stories, I hope to raise awareness of their plight and foster change. The difficulties in their lives are many, and our culture needs to reconsider how to help this group of people with more permanent solutions.

I would like to give tribute and thanks to all the homeless shelters around the world. These are places of hope, healing, kindness, mercy, love and unexpected wisdom. I encourage you to volunteer at one in your neighborhood. You might just meet God there.

ABOUT THE AUTHOR

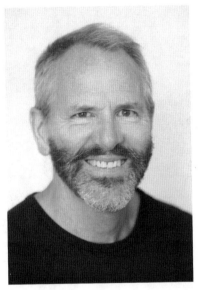

Neil Craton was born and raised in Winnipeg, where he has practiced medicine for 35 years. He has been involved in many aspects of the Winnipeg sport medicine community, including as physician for the Winnipeg Blue Bombers and the Canadian National Women's Volleyball team. Neil serves as a medical educator and is the author of numerous academic works.

ENDNOTES

1. Eugene H. Peterson, *The Message: The Bible in Contemporary Language.* (Colorado Springs: NavPress, 2002) Gal 5:19-*21*

    [19-21] It is obvious what kind of life develops out of trying to get your own way all the time: repetitive, loveless, cheap sex; a stinking accumulation of mental and emotional garbage; frenzied and joyless grabs for happiness; trinket gods; magic-show religion; paranoid loneliness; cutthroat competition; all-consuming-yet-never-satisfied wants; a brutal temper; an impotence to love or be loved; divided homes and divided lives; small-minded and lopsided pursuits; the vicious habit of depersonalizing everyone into a rival; uncontrolled and uncontrollable addictions; ugly parodies of community. I could go on.

2. Benjamin Oldfield and Lauren Small. *The Right to Write About Patients* www.hopkinsmedicine.org Winter 2017.

3. Danielle Ofri, *Adding Spice to the Slog: Humanities in Medical Training.* PloS Med. 2015 Sep; 12(9).

4. Danielle Ofri. *Writing about patients. Is it ethical?* www.huffingtonpost.com May 25, 2011.

5. Scripture quotations are from the HOLY BIBLE, ENGLISH STANDARD VERSION (Wheaton, Good News Publishers, 2007) 2 Corinthians 6:14

^{14} Do not be unequally yoked with unbelievers. For what partnership has righteousness with lawlessness? Or what fellowship has light with darkness?

6. Just as I am (Modern version) Written by: SUE C. SMITH, TRAVIS COTTRELL, DAVID E. MOFFITT Lyrics © Universal Music Publishing Group, CAPITOL CHRISTIAN MUSIC GROUP
   VERSE 1:
   Just as I am, without one plea
   But that Thy blood was shed for me
   And that Thou bidst me come to Thee
   O Lamb of God, I come, I come
   CHORUS:
   I come broken to be mended
   I come wounded to be healed
   I come desperate to be rescued
   I come empty to be filled
   I come guilty to be pardoned
   By the blood of Christ the Lamb
   And I'm welcomed with open arms
   Praise God, just as I am
   VERSE 2:
   Just as I am, and waiting not
   To rid my soul of one dark blot
   To Thee whose blood can cleanse each spot
   O Lamb of God, I come, I come
   VERSE 3:
   Just as I am, I would be lost
   But mercy and grace my freedom bought
   And now to glory in Your cross
   Oh Lamb of God I come, I come

7. Eugene H Peterson, *The Message: The Bible in Contemporary Language*. (Colorado Springs: NavPress, 2002).

John 9: 1-11

Walking down the street, Jesus saw a man blind from birth. His disciples asked, "Rabbi, who sinned: this man or his parents, causing him to be born blind?"[3-5] Jesus said, "You're asking the wrong question. You're looking for someone to blame. There is no such cause-effect here. Look instead for what God can do. We need to be energetically at work for the One who sent me here, working while the sun shines. When night falls, the workday is over. For as long as I am in the world, there is plenty of light. I am the world's Light."[6-7] He said this and then spit in the dust, made a clay paste with the saliva, rubbed the paste on the blind man's eyes, and said, "Go, wash at the Pool of Siloam" (Siloam means "Sent"). The man went and washed—and saw.[8] Soon the town was buzzing. His relatives and those who year after year had seen him as a blind man begging were saying, "Why, isn't this the man we knew, who sat here and begged?"[9] Others said, "It's him all right!" But others objected, "It's not the same man at all. It just looks like him." He said, "It's me, the very one."[10] They said, "How did your eyes get opened?"[11] "A man named Jesus made a paste and rubbed it on my eyes and told me, 'Go to Siloam and wash.' I did what he said. When I washed, I saw."

8. Scripture quotations are from the HOLY BIBLE, ENGLISH STANDARD VERSION (Wheaton, Good News Publishers, 2007)

Matthew 9: 35-36 (ESV)

And Jesus went throughout all the cities and villages, teaching in their synagogues and proclaiming the gospel of the kingdom and healing every disease and every affliction. [36] When he saw the crowds, he had compassion for them, because they were harassed and helpless, like sheep without a shepherd.

9. Stephen Gaetz, Erin Dej, Tim Richter, & Melanie Redman (2016): The State of Homelessness in Canada 2016. Toronto: Canadian Observatory on Homelessness Press.

10. Eugene H Peterson, *The Message: The Bible in Contemporary Language.* (Colorado Springs: NavPress, 2002) .

Matthew 25: 31-46. The Sheep and the Goats

[31-33] "When he finally arrives, blazing in beauty and all his angels with him, the Son of Man will take his place on his glorious throne. Then all the nations will be arranged before him and he will sort the people out, much as a shepherd sorts out sheep and goats, putting sheep to his right and goats to his left.

[34-36] "Then the King will say to those on his right, 'Enter, you who are blessed by my Father! Take what's coming to you in this kingdom. It's been ready for you since the world's foundation. And here's why:

I was hungry and you fed me,
I was thirsty and you gave me a drink,
I was homeless and you gave me a room,
I was shivering and you gave me clothes,
I was sick and you stopped to visit,
I was in prison and you came to me.'

[37-40] "Then those 'sheep' are going to say, 'Master, what are you talking about? When did we ever see you hungry and feed you, thirsty and give you a drink? And when did we ever see you sick or in prison and come to you?' Then the King will say, 'I'm telling the solemn truth: Whenever you did one of these things to someone overlooked or ignored, that was me—you did it to me.'

[41-43] "Then he will turn to the 'goats,' the ones on his left, and say, 'Get out, worthless goats! You're good for nothing but the fires of hell. And why? Because—

I was hungry and you gave me no meal,
I was thirsty and you gave me no drink,
I was homeless and you gave me no bed,
I was shivering and you gave me no clothes,
Sick and in prison, and you never visited.'

[44] "Then those 'goats' are going to say, 'Master, what are you talking about? When did we ever see you hungry or thirsty or homeless or shivering or sick or in prison and didn't help?'

[45] "He will answer them, 'I'm telling the solemn truth: Whenever you failed to do one of these things to someone who was being overlooked or ignored, that was me—you failed to do it to me.'

[46] "Then those 'goats' will be herded to their eternal doom, but the 'sheep' to their eternal reward."

11. Scripture taken from the HOLY BIBLE NEW INTERNATIONAL VERSION (Grand Rapids, Zondervan Copyright 1973, 1978, 1984)
Proverbs 23.
Who has woe? Who has sorrow?
Who has strife? Who has complaints?
Who has needless bruises? Who has bloodshot eyes?
Those who linger over wine,
who go to sample bowls of mixed wine.
Do not gaze at wine when it is red,
when it sparkles in the cup,
when it goes down smoothly!
In the end it bites like a snake
and poisons like a viper. Your eyes will see strange sights,
and your mind will imagine confusing things.
You will be like one sleeping on the high seas,
lying on top of the rigging.
"They hit me," you will say, "but I'm not hurt!
They beat me, but I don't feel it!
When will I wake up
so I can find another drink?"

12. Bruce K Alexander. *The Globalization of Addiction. A study in Poverty of the Spirit.* (Oxford University Press, 2008).

13. Scripture taken from the HOLY BIBLE NEW INTERNATIONAL VERSION (Grand Rapids, Zondervan Copyright 1973, 1978, 1984)
Proverbs 16:18 Pride goes before destruction, a haughty spirit before a fall.

14. Scripture taken from the HOLY BIBLE NEW INTERNATIONAL VERSION (Grand Rapids, Zondervan Copyright 1973, 1978, 1984)

Philippians 4 : 6-7 [6] Do not be anxious about anything, but in every situation, by prayer and petition, with thanksgiving, present your requests to God. [7] And the peace of God, which transcends all understanding, will guard your hearts and your minds in Christ Jesus.

15. Scripture taken from the HOLY BIBLE NEW INTERNATIONAL VERSION (Grand Rapids, Zondervan Copyright 1973, 1978, 1984)

Proverbs 16:5. Every one that is proud in heart is an abomination to the Lord: though hand join in hand, he shall not be unpunished.

16. Scripture taken from the HOLY BIBLE NEW INTERNATIONAL VERSION (Grand Rapids, Zondervan Copyright 1973, 1978, 1984)

Luke 15: 11-32 NIV [11] Jesus continued: "There was a man who had two sons. [12] The younger one said to his father, 'Father, give me my share of the estate.' So he divided his property between them.

[13] "Not long after that, the younger son got together all he had, set off for a distant country and there squandered his wealth in wild living. [14] After he had spent everything, there was a severe famine in that whole country, and he began to be in need. [15] So he went and hired himself out to a citizen of that country, who sent him to his fields to feed pigs. [16] He longed to fill his stomach with the pods that the pigs were eating, but no one gave him anything.

[17] "When he came to his senses, he said, 'How many of my father's hired servants have food to spare, and here I am starving to death! [18] I will set out and go back to my father and say to him: Father, I have sinned against heaven and against you. [19] I am no longer worthy to be called your son; make me like one of your hired servants.' [20] So he got up and went to his father.

"But while he was still a long way off, his father saw him and was filled with compassion for him; he ran to his son, threw his arms around him and kissed him.

²¹ "The son said to him, 'Father, I have sinned against heaven and against you. I am no longer worthy to be called your son.'

²² "But the father said to his servants, 'Quick! Bring the best robe and put it on him. Put a ring on his finger and sandals on his feet. ²³ Bring the fattened calf and kill it. Let's have a feast and celebrate. ²⁴ For this son of mine was dead and is alive again; he was lost and is found.' So they began to celebrate.

²⁵ "Meanwhile, the older son was in the field. When he came near the house, he heard music and dancing. ²⁶ So he called one of the servants and asked him what was going on. ²⁷ 'Your brother has come,' he replied, 'and your father has killed the fattened calf because he has him back safe and sound.'

²⁸ "The older brother became angry and refused to go in. So his father went out and pleaded with him. ²⁹ But he answered his father, 'Look! All these years I've been slaving for you and never disobeyed your orders. Yet you never gave me even a young goat so I could celebrate with my friends. ³⁰ But when this son of yours who has squandered your property with prostitutes comes home, you kill the fattened calf for him!'

³¹ "'My son,' the father said, 'you are always with me, and everything I have is yours. ³² But we had to celebrate and be glad, because this brother of yours was dead and is alive again; he was lost and is found.'"

17. Scripture taken from the HOLY BIBLE NEW INTERNATIONAL VERSION (Grand Rapids, Zondervan Copyright 1973, 1978, 1984)

Luke 10: The Good Samaritan

Just then a religion scholar stood up with a question to test Jesus. "Teacher, what do I need to do to get eternal life?"

²⁶ He answered, "What's written in God's Law? How do you interpret it?"

²⁷ He said, "That you love the Lord your God with all your passion and prayer and muscle and intelligence—and that you love your neighbor as well as you do yourself."

²⁸ "Good answer!" said Jesus. "Do it and you'll live."

[29] Looking for a loophole, he asked, "And just how would you define 'neighbor'?"

[30-32] Jesus answered by telling a story. "There was once a man traveling from Jerusalem to Jericho. On the way he was attacked by robbers. They took his clothes, beat him up, and went off leaving him half-dead. Luckily, a priest was on his way down the same road, but when he saw him he angled across to the other side. Then a Levite religious man showed up; he also avoided the injured man.

[33-35] "A Samaritan traveling the road came on him. When he saw the man's condition, his heart went out to him. He gave him first aid, disinfecting and bandaging his wounds. Then he lifted him onto his donkey, led him to an inn, and made him comfortable. In the morning he took out two silver coins and gave them to the innkeeper, saying, 'Take good care of him. If it costs any more, put it on my bill—I'll pay you on my way back.'

[36] "What do you think? Which of the three became a neighbor to the man attacked by robbers?"

[37] "The one who treated him kindly," the religion scholar responded.

Jesus said, "Go and do the same."

18. Truth and Reconciliation Canada. (2015). Honouring the truth, reconciling for the future: Summary of the final report of the Truth and Reconciliation Commission of Canada. Winnipeg: Truth and Reconciliation Commission of Canada.

19. Eugene H. Peterson, *The Message: The Bible in Contemporary Language.* (Colorado Springs: NavPress, 2002) Gospel of John, Chapter 13.

Jesus knew that the Father had put him in complete charge of everything, that he came from God and was on his way back to God. So he got up from the supper table, set aside his robe, and put on an apron. Then he poured water into a basin and began to wash the feet of the disciples, drying them with his apron.

20. Scripture taken from the HOLY BIBLE NEW INTERNATIONAL VERSION (Grand Rapids, Zondervan Copyright 1973, 1978, 1984) Matthew 20: 20-28.

Then the mother of Zebedee's sons came to Jesus with her sons and, kneeling down, asked a favor of him.

21 "What is it you want?" he asked.

She said, "Grant that one of these two sons of mine may sit at your right and the other at your left in your kingdom."

22 "You don't know what you are asking," Jesus said to them. "Can you drink the cup I am going to drink?"

"We can," they answered.

23 Jesus said to them, "You will indeed drink from my cup, but to sit at my right or left is not for me to grant. These places belong to those for whom they have been prepared by my Father."

24 When the ten heard about this, they were indignant with the two brothers. 25 Jesus called them together and said, "You know that the rulers of the Gentiles lord it over them, and their high officials exercise authority over them. 26 Not so with you. Instead, whoever wants to become great among you must be your servant, 27 and whoever wants to be first must be your slave—28 just as the Son of Man did not come to be served, but to serve, and to give his life as a ransom for many."

21. air07. Justice, Mercy and Grace. Thetruthspeakproject.wordpress.com. August 19, 2011

22. Denny Bellesi and Leesa Bellesi, *The Kingdom Assignment – What will you do with the talents God has given you?* (Grand Rapids: Zondervan, 2001)

23. Scripture taken from the HOLY BIBLE NEW INTERNATIONAL VERSION (Grand Rapids, Zondervan Copyright 1973, 1978, 1984) Romans 5: 1-5 Therefore, since we have been justified through faith, we[a] have peace with God through our Lord Jesus Christ, 2 through whom we have gained access by faith into this grace in which we now

stand. And we[b] boast in the hope of the glory of God. [3] Not only so, but we[c] also glory in our sufferings, because we know that suffering produces perseverance; [4] perseverance, character; and character, hope. [5] And hope does not put us to shame, because God's love has been poured out into our hearts through the Holy Spirit, who has been given to us.

24. Leah Denbok. *Nowhere to Call Home. Photographs and Stories of the Homeless. Volume One* (Victoria, FriesenPress) 2017.

Printed in Canada